2/13

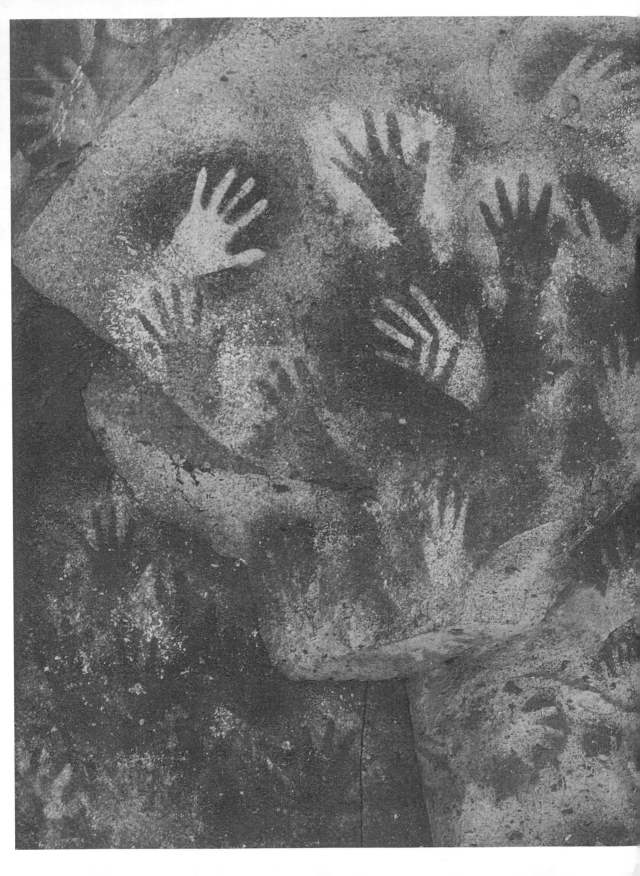

THE
PRIMAL
CONNECTION

MARK SISSON

THE PRIMAL CONNECTION

Library of Congress Control Number: 2012920049
Library of Congress Cataloging-in-Publication Data is on file with the publisher
Sisson, Mark, 1953–

The Primal Connection: Follow Your Genetic Blueprint to Health and Happiness / Mark Sisson

ISBN: 9780984755103
1. Self-help 2. Health&Fitness 3. Body, Mind & Spirit

Editor/Project Manager: Jessica Taylor Tudzin
Design/Layout and Illustrations: Caroline De Vita
Writing/Research: Jennifer Zotalis, Brad Kearns
Copy Editor: Nancy Wong Bryan
Editorial Assistant: Nancy Lehigh, Elizabeth Kane
Back Cover Photo: Tahia Hocking
Indexing: Leoni McVey

Content and images on the Gokhale Method was sourced from *8 Steps to a Healthy Back* with permission from the author, Esther Gokhale.

For more information about the Primal Blueprint,
please visit primalblueprint.com.
For information on quantity discounts, please call 888-774-6259

Publisher: Primal Blueprint Publishing.
23805 Stuart Ranch Rd. Suite 145 Malibu, CA 90265

CONTENTS

DISCLAIMER

THE IDEAS, CONCEPTS AND OPINIONS expressed in this book are intended to be used for educational purposes only. This book is sold with the understanding that author and publisher are not rendering medical advice of any kind, nor is this book intended to replace medical advice, nor to diagnose, prescribe or treat any disease, condition, illness or injury. It is imperative that before beginning any diet or exercise program, including any aspect of the Primal Blueprint program, you receive full medical clearance from a licensed physician. Author and publisher claim no responsibility to any person or entity for any liability, loss, or damage caused or alleged to be caused directly or indirectly as a result of the use, application or interpretation of the material in this book. If you object to this disclaimer, you may return the book to the publisher for a full refund.

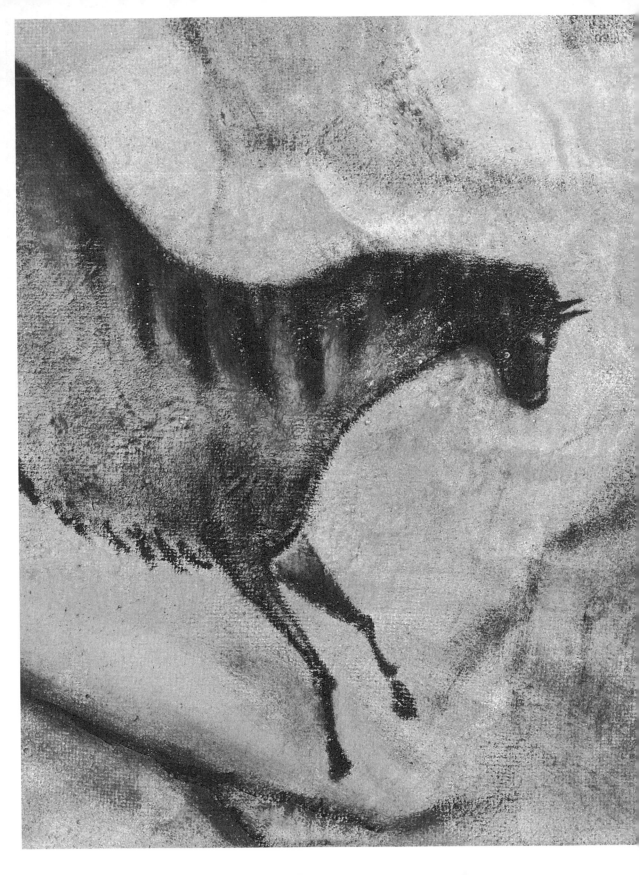

INTRODUCTION

There is more wisdom in your body than
in your deepest philosophies.

FRIEDRICH NIETZSCHE

WELCOME TO
THE PRIMAL CONNECTION

AN ADVANCE NOTICE: THIS IS not a book about living a more gracious life. Nor is it written to stir sentimentality or foster sophistication. On the contrary, it's an endeavor best undertaken with sleeves rolled up. Prepare to get your hands dirty. We'll be digging down to the rudiments. It's about unearthing something in ourselves that has been lost, buried, or obscured. It's about reconnecting with the less acknowledged, let alone less appreciated, layers of ourselves. It's about getting to the very essence of what makes us human and tapping into our genetic recipe for health, happiness, and fulfillment.

You see, I know many people who are by all normal measures of society considered "successful." In some cases, they have accomplished a great deal professionally. Many have families. All have a significant circle of close friends. Still, they often speak of a nebulous, hollow feeling. It's as if something is missing, as if they have forgotten some important aspect of life somewhere along the way. They often describe a sense of emptiness, of not feeling truly *connected*—at least not in the way that has them jumping out of bed to greet every day with enthusiasm. In many cases this void is nothing more than a minor distraction, a simple intuitive sense that maybe there's something more to life, or maybe there's something they're not doing right.

They try to fill the void in different ways: enrolling in a new class, attending church, volunteering, or taking up philanthropy. You may relate. We are bombarded daily with magazines, TV shows, and self-help books offering plenty of "healthy living" directives—take this pill, take this vacation, take advantage of this special offer, run this 26.2-mile race, follow this eating regimen, and so on. While these suggestions can certainly help unburden the psyche, they fail to address the core issue—just as taking a blood thinner fails to address the actual cause of a blocked artery. The emptiness goes deeper. It's more innate, more instinctual, more organic. It's something untapped.

Many people take medications to better deal with the turbulent times—filling prescriptions for anxiety, depression, or insomnia—often for good reason, but in some cases with misgivings. Some seek out the advice of therapists or life coaches to help them. They delve into old memories, past intentions, trying to heal childhood wounds, all in hopes of feeling better, feeling more alive.

In an age of distractions, relentless stress, strained relationships, and overemphasized materialism, we often try to rationalize our way toward some precipitous point of balance. We follow regimens. We manage our time and relationships. We pencil in physical activities. We compartmentalize our needs and anxieties. For all the comforts and conveniences, the innovations and accommodations, something about this whole picture of modern living isn't working for us. For all our knowledge, we impose an increasingly narrow, shallow definition on wellbeing.

So, what makes for a healthy, grounded life, anyway? What does it genuinely mean to thrive, to feel satisfied and fulfilled? We assume the answers are to be found in further progress: a new medication, a more elaborate gadget, the latest fitness class, or a social trend. The truth is, the answers we seek are often not that complicated.

What if it isn't a failure of progress but the frustration of some unmet need at the cellular level? What if we entertain the notion that we aren't—all of us as a hominid species—living the lives we were designed to live? Forget the caves and skins and matted hair for a minute. I'm talking about a life of physical challenge but ample leisure. I'm talking about living by the natural ebb and flow of light and darkness, season to season. I'm talking about living in smaller groups. I'm talking about play and creativity and getting dirt under our fingernails—a life of the raw senses and an overlapping of the self and the natural environment.

I've been thinking about human health—researching and writing about it—for some thirty years now. My initial explorations into what it means to be healthy and fit centered on my own failings as an endurance athlete. I had blindly followed conventional wisdom to sculpt myself into the most race-fit human possible, yet as I worked toward that goal I simultaneously became injured and ill. "What's wrong with this picture?" I asked myself.

After an early forced retirement, I vowed to find ways to become the healthy, strong, lean, and fit person I always wanted to be ... but without having to struggle and sacrifice so much to get there. I truly believed I could have it all, and that getting there did not have to be as difficult as most of us make it out to be. The convergence of modern genetic science and evolutionary biology led me to an ancestral approach to health and fitness. A pattern emerged. If we could eat and move like our ancestors did—within the context of a convenient, high-tech, and sometimes hedonistic twenty-first-century existence—then we would experience optimal health. It was as if our genes expect us to live a certain way, and we, through progress and convenience, have forgotten how to do that.

It makes intuitive sense that the foods our species has been eating over the longest span of time are also the foods to which we are most highly adapted. It makes intuitive sense that the movements we've been performing for the longest time are also movements which our bodies perform best and which elicit the most favorable hormonal responses or gene expression. After making a few simple adjustments to my diet and exercise routine, my health improved. This became the lifeway I started calling the Primal Blueprint, which I write about extensively on my blog, Mark's Daily Apple.

In researching and writing my 2009 book, *The Primal Blueprint*, I quickly began to grasp what I believe to be the single most empowering fact of our lives: that we all possess the genetic recipe to build a strong, lean, fit, happy, healthy, loving, productive, fulfilled human being. The process by which we each fulfill that recipe, however, is largely up to the choices each one of us makes. Sure, some of us are taller, some bigger, some faster, some slightly more predisposed to diabetes or arthritis. Our parental genes determine such unchangeable variances in our genetic makeup—they provide the *range of possible outcomes within the basic genetic recipe* to build a human being. That basic recipe, however, is the same for all of us. Each of us metabolizes food, stores and burns fat, builds muscle, heals wounds, and carries out almost every biological process using the same biochemistry—it's simply the degree to which our bodies do these things that determines the difference.

That diet and exercise are ways in which we can harness gene expression to rebuild, renew, and regenerate ourselves every moment is obvious to me. But in a short time, I came to believe that there was much more to uncover. Maybe we are wired for happiness and contentment just as we are for fitness and health. I started thinking about sunlight, how I'd always felt better when I had a bit of a tan going, and how sunny days are invariably happy days. Why is that? Maybe there was something happening to our neurochemistry as a result. Maybe it wasn't just psychological.

Thus began my exploration into how we live today and connecting it with research about our primal ancestors. As with diet and exercise, it seemed perfectly logical that our bodies have come to *expect* certain environmental inputs such as exposure to sunlight and darkness, both of which regulate our sleep habits based on millions of years of environmental pressures. (Ahh, so it was no small coincidence then that maintaining a modest year-round tan made me feel healthy and happy.)

From there, I began exploring how all the other environmental factors in our evolutionary ancestors' lives may have shaped them ... and us. As far as I was concerned, everything was fair game. What else could we learn from our ancestors' habitude? What more could we gain from understanding the evolutionary legacy that lives in each of us?

Moving away from the trappings and stresses of modern life is one of, if not the, key goal in the Primal Blueprint approach. However, when our relationship with our primal ancestors gets distilled into just how we diet and exercise, we lose sight of that ultimate goal. Considering that our more advanced natures have been evolving over some two million years, what else might our genes expect from our environment? Specific sleep conditions? Certain models of socialization? Interaction with nature? Play? Beyond these questions of what, there's the question of *how* these inclinations unfold in modern humans in a modern world. Are we meeting them? How do our innate expectations conflict with our contemporary lifestyles?

I began writing about environmental factors on Mark's Daily Apple, comparing our ancestral settings and activities with those of today, citing current and compelling research, and offering up concrete ideas for reclaiming—with modern adaptations—pivotal elements of our primal origins.

Readers told me I was opening up whole new dimensions to *The Primal Blueprint*. It was becoming, in their encouraging words, a broader, deeper design for them in achieving a richer, more fulfilling, as well as physically healthier life. I found the same benefits in living out these new principles, which I started calling the Primal Connection, in my own life. If we view every aspect of our lives through an evolutionary lens, we find perspective in the choices we make. Often it provides more options—some quite surprising. *The Primal Connection*, I believe, can do for our psyches what *The Primal Blueprint* has done for many people's physical health.

Over the course of the last few years, readers have shared their stories of implementing the Primal Connection vision. And in no uncertain terms, they told me they wanted more. Mark's Daily Apple readers were the first to encourage me to write this book, and I thank them for the incredible enthusiasm and extraordinary insights that helped inspire it. This book is the culmination—and a reflection—of years of research and continuing conversations with readers and experts in fields as diverse as medicine, psychology, anthropology, and neurology.

The essential underlying premise of *The Primal Connection* journey is this: the more we live like our evolutionary ancestors, the healthier we are, the more efficient our physiological functioning, the more normalized our hormonal responses, the more health promoting our epigenetic storyline ... and quite likely, the more content, satisfied, and fulfilled we can be. We're about to discover and tap into the power of our genetic coding, what I like to call our factory settings, to understand and exploit (with practical modern adaptation) the default expectations genetically developed over the arc of our evolutionary history. The concept of ancestral archetype makes intuitive—even elegant—sense. It also bears out under the harsh light of scientific inquiry. There's no proposal in this book that doesn't jibe with contemporary research.

You will notice a few recurring themes as this book unfolds. The first is that our genes expect certain inputs and behaviors from us. When we generally "stick to the script" and provide the kinds of inputs our genes have evolved to expect over millennia, they get the signal to build or to regenerate us as healthy, strong, happy people. That's what our DNA recipe calls for. When we don't provide the expected inputs, our genes still take action, but in this case are often signaled to take steps to protect us from short-term harm in ways that compromise long-term health. For example, we carry around excess body fat because our genes—forged in a crucible of carbohydrate scarcity—now experience carbohydrate overabundance. This causes our fat-storing, sugar-burning genes to up-regulate, and our fat-burning genes to down-regulate. Type 2 diabetes, then, isn't so much an example of weak or defective genes as it is a condition wherein our perfect human genes are attempting to protect us from an excess sugar intake and a lifetime of poor diet and exercise choices.

This brings us to the second theme: we live in a world where abundance and scarcity are often mismatched with what our genes expect. We now have abundant access to all sorts of sugars (grains, alcohol, refined sugar, and fruit year-round), comforts and conveniences (electricity, automobiles, refrigeration, climate control, digital gadgets, and so forth), and instant and passive gratification (drugs, porn, reality TV, Facebook, and so on). All this was either extremely scarce or completely nonexistent until most recently in our evolutionary timeline.

On the flip side, what was once abundant—leisure time, participation in nature, sun exposure, natural sound cues, for example—is now scarce. If we do bring these things into our lives, it's now by conscious, deliberate choice. Naturally, problems arise as a result of these mismatches, affecting our genes, hormones, neurotransmitters, receptors, and other biological processes that were all originally developed under the selection pressure of scarcity and threat of death. Though the primitive threats to our survival no longer exist in most places on the globe today, our genetic hardwiring still expects—and actually appreciates—a certain measure of scarcity for some things and a certain measure of abundance for others.

The third theme you will see throughout this book is what I call "chasing the high." That is, making choices that seem like a good idea at the time, but ultimately backfire to our detriment. I'm referring to self-stimulating our innate, survival-driven, feel-good hormonal reward system to the point of excess or addiction, usually the result of overindulging in stimuli that once were exceptionally scarce or nonexistent. We might overeat carbs for quick energy and a pulse of serotonin, or become addicted to drugs, sex, gambling, texting, or even long-distance running for the feel-good endorphins and opioids. Each time we are rewarded, we come back for more. We aren't at all unlike Pavlov's dogs in that regard. It indeed behooves us to engage our higher-level reasoning and evaluate the long-term consequences of short-term gratification.

But let's be perfectly clear. I'm not advocating a return to the caves, and, for the record, I'm not out to confiscate anyone's iPhone. This is not about abandoning modern society or donning skins and living in the wilderness. (If that's your thing, however, go for it.) *The Primal Connection* is about infusing our modern lives with the best and most reasonably reclaimed elements of our evolutionary past, including time outdoors, all-consuming play, human touch, and deeper social connections, for the simple purpose of making us happier, healthier, and well adjusted. It's about simplifying, stripping away layers of complexity, giving yourself a break, reframing your perspective, and lowering your stress levels by acting, breathing, moving, and thinking in ways that promote optimal gene expression. There is no requirement to master intensive study topics, allocate massive amounts of time to a long list of daily to-do items, or eschew most of the pleasures and comforts we enjoy in modern life. You will see plenty of suggestions and directives to implement each connection, but personal preference, and your own sense of what resonates, will dictate how you express them. What's key is that your intention—and your will to take action—is pure. But before you jump in, let's take a look at the connections you are about to explore:

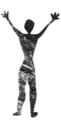 **THE INNER DIALOGUE CONNECTION.** This section will address our inner chatter—the monologues, diatribes, and even full dialogues we carry on within our heads. The majority of the monkey chatter we manufacture in our minds is negative self-talk: obsessing about superficial concerns, worry over the imagined outcome of events that have yet to (and likely may never) happen. In the Inner Dialogue Connection, you will learn the 10 Habits of Highly Successful Hunter-Gatherers, including taking responsibility for your life, being present, trusting your gut, mastering your skills, and redefining your concept of affluence.

THE BODY CONNECTION. In this section, you will learn how the silent, potent language of human touch positively affects us on the biochemical level, providing comfort and healing. You'll learn why wearing shoes can cause lower back pain, skewed postural alignment, and impaired hip mobility, and how going barefoot will not only reduce or eliminate such ailments, but help build a strong Achilles tendon and improve your posture. Speaking of which, did you know that a J-shaped spine is more natural to the human form than the S-shaped spine promoted by conventional wisdom? We'll look closer at the biomechanics of posture and moving, and discuss why taking frequent breaks and moving frequently throughout the day provides more health benefits than just a single one-hour daily workout.

 THE NATURE CONNECTION. You'll find that spending time in nature is not just a refreshing sensory escape, but a necessary balance to the distractions of the modern world. Even if you're firmly rooted in an urban jungle, you can give your genes the nature experience they expect, even if that means some of it is simulated through imagery and recorded sounds. And you'll learn to express your primal need to claim your habitat by navigating your home surroundings on foot. You'll learn why getting dirty—through gardening or having a mud fight with the neighborhood kids—can dramatically boost mood, cognition, and immune function (and why you will want to temper your clean-freak tendencies).

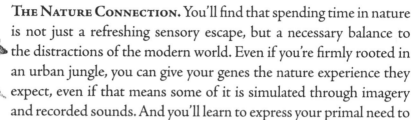 **THE DAILY RHYTHM CONNECTION.** For more than 2.5 million years of human history, the solar sequence of daybreak and nightfall has indelibly imprinted our gene pattern with hormone and biochemical releases that trigger our sleep, wakefulness, and activity levels. Our conquest over light and dark with artificial illumination overrides this natural circadian rhythm. To accommodate to the constructs of society, day and night are now contrived lengths, demanding of us shorter sleep cycles and longer periods of wakefulness. Add the barrage of media, technology, and communication that must be filtered and managed today, and our already distorted, biological cadence is decidedly off-tempo, degrading our health and wellbeing. You will learn ways to counteract the data storm, reset your circadian clock to a closer replica of your genetic model, and slow down.

THE SOCIAL CONNECTION. We are all looking for ways to maximize quality time with our closest friends and family in the midst of the daily demands that are placed on us. This section will discuss the health benefits of building and

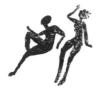maintaining close social ties, consider the influx of social media, and question if we are hardwired to interact within small groups rather than manage larger groups numbering in the hundreds. You will be challenged to look at the superficial connections that eat away at your time and energy, and reassess and prioritize the people of most importance in your life. And finally, you will learn ways to walk through the mindless electronic chatter to more personal, peaceful, and satisfying social relationships.

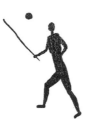**THE PLAY CONNECTION.** The need for play doesn't go away as we grow up; it actually becomes more necessary the more complex our lives become. Play was a vital part of primal life, helping our ancestors experiment, problem solve, and increase knowledge without having to face real-life (or death!) pressures. True play is commonly neglected these days in favor of artificial, leisure-time fillers—computer, TV, digital games, Facebook—that do little or nothing toward refreshing or re-orienting us, or enriching our relationships. The innocent fun of childhood can be ours again, especially with outdoor activity. Adult playtime will help break you out of your regimented daily routine and awaken your creativity and fun-loving spirit. We'll explore a raft of artistic and athletic possibilities to consider.

At this time, I'd like to make the ambitious assumption that you are familiar with the Primal Blueprint philosophy as it relates to the basics of eating and exercise. As we venture beyond what's on your dinner plate to discuss the thoughts in your head, the feelings in your heart, and the social customs of daily life as they relate to optimal gene expression, I must assert that the gateway this book offers to happiness and contentment will be more easily accessible if you are practicing the movement's basic principles. If you are falling short of optimal eating and exercise, it's best to take a few steps back and acquaint yourself with the basics before contemplating the higher levels of awareness offered in this book.

THE PRIMAL BLUEPRINT DIET AND EXERCISE AT A GLANCE

Eat Primal Foods. Meat, fish, fowl, eggs, vegetables, fruits, nuts, and seeds are nutritious, highly satisfying, and promote stabilized energy levels and efficient burning of stored body fat for energy.

Ditch Toxic Modern Foods. The excessive intake of processed carbohydrates and chemically altered fats in the Standard American Diet (SAD) may be the most health-destructive element of modern life. Excess insulin production from a high-carbohydrate diet leads to burnout, fatigue, disease, lifelong weight gain, and a continued dependency on additional health-compromising carbs! Eliminate the following SAD staples:

- **Sugars and sweetened beverages:** Consumption of processed sweets that our genes are not accustomed to promotes wildly excessive insulin production, suppresses immune function, and accelerates aging.
- **Grains:** Wheat, corn, rice, cereal, pasta, and all derivatives such as breads, crackers, energy bars, breakfast staples, pizza, chips, cooking grains, and packaged snacks. Yep, even whole grains are troublesome, stimulating excessinsulin production and containing antinutrients that compromise digestion and immune function.
- **Vegetable oils:** These promote free-radical damage and accelerate aging. Toss them out and stick with butter for cooking.
- **Processed and packaged foods:** If it's in a box or a wrapper, far from a state found in nature, think twice.

Exercise Primally. An increase in everyday activity—including low-intensity aerobic workouts (walking, hiking, easy cycling, cardio machines, jogging) and intense (but brief) sprints and strength training—will optimize fat metabolism, delay the aging process, build and maintain lean muscle mass, and develop lifelong functional fitness. Avoid the prevailing chronic approach to exercise, where workouts are too hard, too lengthy, too frequent, and do not allow sufficient rest in between. With the Primal approach, maximum results can be achieved with minimal time and suffering!

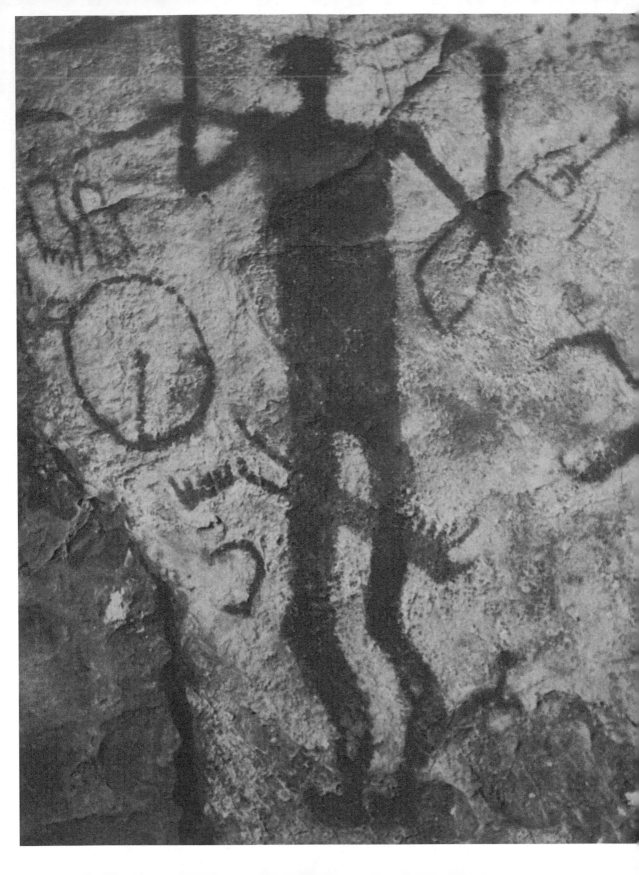

A Recipe For Success

As a product of millions of years of evolutionary design, you are hardwired to feel good. When our evolutionary ancestors ate, slept, touched, loved, hunted, and played, they were rewarded with the release of adaptive "feel good" hormones and neurotransmitters—oxytocin, dopamine, endorphins, and serotonin, to name a few. Repeating behaviors that made us feel good advanced the goals of evolution—that is, to survive and pass on our genetic material to the next generation. Genetically speaking, we are still identical to our hunter-gatherer ancestors so these behaviors remain universal. Though we are unchanged, our world is not. Scarcity has given way to overabundance, and vice versa. As a result, instead of facing the selection pressures of predators and starvation, our danger now lies in self-stimulating our feel-good hormones by artificial or excessive means. Indeed, our innate reward system can either act to our detriment when we abuse it, or act as an inner compass that can lead us toward better health, peace of mind, short-term pleasure, and long-term happiness.

The genes are the bricks and mortar to build a brain.
The environment is the architect.

CHRISTINE HOHMANN
NEUROSCIENTIST

HARDWIRED FOR FEEL-GOOD HORMONES

WE HUMANS ARE HARDWIRED TO pursue pleasure. No doubt, you've long been aware that whenever you exercise, eat nutritious food, have sex, spend time in nature, align your sleep habits with the sun, and foster supportive relationships, you feel pretty darn good. You feel energized, positive, excited, motivated, loving, powerful, fulfilled, and happy. This built-in reward system represents the essence of survival. It acts as an inner compass that guides you to pursue social, geographical, cultural, nutritional, and physical behaviors that reward on a biochemical level, all the way from such basic needs as acquiring shelter, food, and safety, on up the list to more refined endeavors such as pondering ethical dilemmas, pursuing creative outlets, and engaging high-level reasoning. Fact is, whenever we do anything that confers a survival benefit to our species, we reinforce ancient neural pathways and produce feel-good hormones and neurochemicals.

Of course, this flies in the face of the behaviorist school of thought, which operates on the implicit assumption that we come into this world as "blank slates," empty pages upon which we personally compose our life narratives. Yes, it's true that we make an infinite number of active and (hopefully) conscious choices that help direct our life's course. Yet, as evolutionary psychologist Steven Pinker and other scientific experts tell us, that's only part of the story.

We come into this world as products—and bearers—of millions of years of evolutionary design. Many of the attributes, motivations, and anxieties that characterize our individual lives today have their roots in experiences from thousands, even millions, of years ago. These are what I refer to throughout this book as the expectations of our hunter-gatherer genes—the DNA "recipe" for a healthy, fit, happy, loving human. There are certain inputs our *Homo sapiens sapiens* genes anticipate and expect based on evolution. When we don't provide those inputs, we develop disconnects that can lead to disease and depression.

> **Many of the attributes, motivations, and anxieties that characterize our individual lives today have their roots in experiences from thousands, even millions, of years ago.**

The long road of evolution shaped how our bodies developed—walking upright and having opposable thumbs, for instance. It also shaped how our brains developed and, with it, the emotional states and cognitive heights we're capable of experiencing. In recent years, with the study of *epigenetics*, we've begun looking at how our environment and activities turn on and turn off certain genes to affect our cells positively or adversely. It is incredibly empowering to realize the impact simple lifestyle choices can have on health, maybe even despite the familial genetic hand you personally may have been dealt.

The popular concept of *genes* is that they are simply static sequences of DNA that determine hereditary traits, behaviors, and predispositions such as eye, skin, or hair color, or the tendency to reach a certain height or weight. In terms of risk factors for certain diseases, if you inherit the "gene for breast cancer," for example,

MEET GROK:
Those familiar with The Primal Blueprint *and MarksDailyApple.com know Grok, my nickname for the prototypical pre-agricultural human being who lived some ten thousand years ago.*

it's assumed that you're going to get breast cancer. There's some element of truth that one's heredity may confer a higher risk; however, that's an overly simplified explanation. In reality, genes are not traits; genes must be *expressed* in order to trigger the traits for which they are coded. This is called *gene expression*.

When a gene is expressed, it produces a protein called a *gene product*. Gene products are the real agents in genetics and in life and, depending on which gene produced it, a gene product can have any number of effects on the organism in which it resides. Think of the changes you see in a growing child. Gene

> **Genes are not traits; genes must be *expressed* in order to trigger the traits for which they are coded. This is called *gene expression*.**

expression is responsible for creating the gene products that instruct that child's bones to grow—and how much to grow. It's through gene expression that the genotype (the genetic recipe that is similar in all humans, but is unique to each of us in terms of hereditary information) leads to the phenotype (the observable properties expressed by way of behavior, appearance, growth, and disease). Genes represent potential. Gene products realize—or don't realize—that potential. Everything that makes us who we are is controlled through gene expression.

Epigenetics explains how controllable environmental factors—the food you eat, the sleep you get, the exercise you do, the amount of sunlight you're exposed to, the social interactions you have, even the thoughts you think or how much you laugh at a joke—trigger gene expression in different biochemical ways. What this means is that your genes are not your destiny, that you have the power to control the way your genes are turned on and off by your behaviors and lifestyle. By learning about these hidden genetic switches and the epigenetic inputs that affect them, you can affect your health and your sense of wellbeing.

In order for an epigenetic input to bring about gene expression, we need a messenger. Enter *hormones*, chemicals released from our cells and glands to deliver much of this epigenetic data to our genes. When the information arrives at the gene, hormones interact with hormone receptors, and this interaction helps decide how the gene will be expressed. In effect, hormones relay environmental inputs to our genes so that they can produce the gene product required for a proper response. Most of the hormonal interaction our genes experience happens at the subconscious level, but sometimes we can actually *feel* the effects of hormones because they interact with genes that affect behavior and subjective experience. Goose bumps, anyone?

If hormones are the long-distance messengers, then *neurotransmitters* are the local messengers. In the brain, neurotransmitters deliver similar information from one neuron to another. Neurons have neurotransmitter receptors, and certain neurotransmitters have different effects on the neurons that receive them. Some are *excitatory* neurotransmitters, meaning they increase the chance the target neuron will fire and be active, while others are *inhibitory* neurotransmitters, meaning they decrease the chance the target neuron will fire and be active. It is through neurotransmitters that the neurons communicate with each other, relaying emotions and memories as well as signaling how to interpret raw sensory data. Let's take a closer look at how some common environmental inputs can have epigenetic effects on your genome:

When you laugh[1] or immerse yourself in natural settings such as a forest,[2] the genes that control your natural killer cells (NK cells)—an important part of your innate immune system that defends against infections, cancer, and other pathogens—are turned on and expressed. It's worth noting that NK cells also help regulate blood sugar. In fact, people with type 2 diabetes can lower their blood sugar after a meal just by enjoying a good laugh.

Clean freaks of the world should note that digging your hands into soil stimulates increased levels of serotonin, a mood-elevating neurotransmitter that also plays a major role in the regulation of your sleep, appetite, and cognitive performance. When your body is exposed to *M. vaccae* and other bacteria contained in dirt, your immune system is prompted to release cytokines, the protein messengers that signal the release of serotonin. The hygiene hypothesis, which I will cover in detail in the Nature Connection, proposes that exposure to dirt and other unpolluted, organic matter will improve your immune system and brain function.

The simple act of another person touching you can reduce the stress hormone cortisol by expressing the gene that controls the cortisol receptor.[3] When the receptor is expressed, it absorbs the cortisol and thus reduces its destructive effects. Touch also expresses the OXT gene,[4] which encodes for oxytocin delivery, an "empathy" hormone that increases trust, allows emotional connections, and moderates cortisol.

Then there is vitamin D, which is actually not a vitamin but a powerful hormone—one of the body's most important—that interacts with the hundreds of genes necessary for health and survival. When you spend time in the sun, your skin synthesizes vitamin D in response to UVB rays. The vitamin D hormone in turn expresses the gene POMC that *protects* against melanoma.[5] (You read

> ❝ **None of us could get through a day without using the rational, directed attention the neocortex provides.** ❞

that right. Moderate sunlight—contrary to conventional wisdom—protects you from the most serious form of skin cancer.) POMC, or pro-opiomelanocortin, also creates the opioid peptides that make the warm sun feel so good on our skin. James Watson, the father of modern genetic science who co-discovered the double helix in 1953, identified this gene as his favorite of all twenty-thousand-plus human genes, telling *Forbes* magazine in a 2012 interview that its very structure is an implicit biological message. "Happiness is a reward for doing what we should be doing," he said. "For being in the sun and making vitamin D, for exercising, and for bringing nutrients into our bodies."

Vitamin D also expresses the BGLAP gene, which is encoded to produce osteocalcin, the compound that builds and strengthens bone. It interacts with IRF8, a gene that appears to thwart multiple sclerosis, and with PTPN2, a gene linked to preventing type 1 diabetes, Crohn's disease, and virtually all autoimmune diseases.[6] Without adequate vitamin D, however, these protective genes cannot be expressed, and the risk of rickets, osteoporosis, multiple sclerosis, and autoimmune disease increases dramatically. And that's just a small snippet of the range of genes that vitamin D helps to express. Hundreds more, ranging from genes that control blood lipid levels to genes that influence height, all depend on adequate amounts of vitamin D. Imagine that—a little bit of sunlight can help determine all those essential aspects of health that many of us assumed were out of our control!

We can thank a class of pleasure-giving neurotransmitters called opioid peptides for encouraging us to seek out epigenetic inputs that improve our survival. According to Kent Berridge, a neuroscientist at the University of Michigan, this is probably true of all pleasures. Here's Berridge:

> In the past ten years, a body of evidence shows all the pleasures we experience produce activity in the same brain systems. For example, the nucleus accumbens activates to intensely pleasant music, winning money, and seeing a loved one, just as it activates to food or drug sensory pleasures.[7]

In other words, things don't just feel good for no reason. There's always an explanation for it couched in gene expression.

In terms of how our brains operate, we will be looking primarily at two modes of thinking in *The Primal Connection*—"top down" and "bottom up." Our predominant mode of thinking is top down, which works in a controlled, rationalistic way that involves lining up and fitting details into a preconceived project or assumption. For example, ticking items off your to-do list or applying highly specialized work skills. It's actually called "top down" because the area of the brain involved—the neocortex—is located behind the forehead at the brain's forefront, i.e., the top. This is the part of the brain that gives us the ability to process what-if scenarios, and is one of the more advanced developments of our species.

The frontal lobe, however, works best when balanced with input from the cerebellum (Latin for *little brain*), one of the most primal parts of the brain, second to the brainstem itself and located at the back of your head, i.e., the bottom. We sometimes call it the "lizard brain" for its role in reactive motor control, fear, and pleasure responses. This is the part of the brain that also processes sensory awareness, also known as involuntary attention.

None of us could get through a day without using the rational, directed attention the neocortex provides. This sort of thinking benefited our Paleolithic ancestors, allowing them to create all manner of early technology, language, and culture. It becomes an issue, however, when it predominates our lives. Not only does the brain tire of focusing in this mode for prolonged periods, but we end up missing out on the creative, emotional, and restorative advantages of a more primary means of encountering the world. When we turn our attention to sensory awareness—"bottom up" cognition—we release the filters and expectations we so often put in the way of living. Although we derive the benefit of involuntary attention in other settings, natural settings are the original and perhaps richest model for entering this state.

Though the feel-good behaviors—the connections—covered in *The Primal Connection* are universal, the ways in which each of us satisfies them are not. As the twentieth-century behaviorist B.F. Skinner's theory of operant conditioning assumes, your behavior is driven by a unique set of *psychological mechanisms* that respond to a history of reinforcement—both positive and negative—that you have experienced in your life. According to this view, psychological mechanisms are a product of nurture and environment, and are constantly evolving.

For instance, let's say you have a positive experience surfing in the ocean, tending to your garden, or listening to hip-hop music. You are likely compelled to pursue the experience again and again, and with good reason. On the other hand, you try to avoid those experiences that you associate with stress, pain, and discomfort, unless you perceive some form of payoff that outweighs the negative associations. Suppose you associate the beach with too much sun and wind. You likely won't go. But the fact remains that you will still have a deep-seated need to experience nature, so you might find other ways to satisfy your genetic expectations, maybe up in the mountains or in a rainforest. Either that, or you'll frustrate your genes entirely!

The point is—and this is where the science of epigenetics intersects with Skinner's behavioral psychology—we all have basic, hardwired requirements for health, balance, and happiness. We are all preprogrammed to interact with nature, to seek downtime for solitude and silence, to socialize with a smaller group of people than what populates our Facebook list, to get up and move throughout the day. However, the particulars of how you or I or anyone else satisfies these needs can and do vary wildly. Such is the spice of life and the power of personal preference. Don't let any diet guru, life coach, or any other impure influence try to tell you differently. No one knows better how to float your boat than you.

Take music, for example. A human being's emotional makeup is innately designed to respond to musical sounds and rhythms. Charles Darwin, among other theorists, believed that the earliest forms of music imitated primitive animal cries. Primal cultures emulated those sounds to control pain, induce trances, and attract mates. Today, music has evolved to become more structured and varied, which is to say if hip-hop doesn't resonate with you, you can call up a classical or country-western piece and experience the same biochemical benefits as the guy with the low, baggy jeans rockin' out to his beat. Indeed, studies show that music helps reduce stress as well as improve cognition and memory function—and it doesn't matter what kind of music it is, as long as you enjoy it. At its basic level it's still just neurotransmitters and hormones providing feedback and signaling gene expression.

"" If you go through life in a steady state of homeostasis, you tend to atrophy, not just muscularly but hormonally as well. ""

We know we are happiest when we are free to explore life, liberty, and the pursuit of happiness. The problem is modern life's busyness and incongruence with the evolutionary model leaves us struggling, quite frequently, to even picture what a truly healthy, grounded life looks like. In our frenetic, go-go-go, produce-at-all-costs world, perhaps you envision it as a constant state of homeostasis, where all systems in your body are stable and in balance. No doubt, a healthy mind and body depend on equilibrium.

However, it is possible to have too much of a good thing. Live a life of too much ease and comfort (or just plain boredom), and your hormones get locked into a way of operating, essentially "forgetting" their purpose, that is, to respond to life-threatening, life-jolting events. If you go through life in a steady state of homeostasis, you tend to atrophy, not just muscularly but hormonally as well. Indeed, even at the gene level we operate under one of nature's most basic principles: use it or lose it. If a process takes energy (a scarce commodity for most of our evolution), and you're not currently using that process for survival, epigenetic signals usually allow the genes to "down-regulate" or turn off that system. You would be well served, then, to identify which systems in your body have been neglected and address any deficiency according to the guidelines offered within this book.

Life for our ancestors was a lot like war is now: long periods of boredom interrupted by brief moments of terror. They lived with a tremendous amount of slow-paced downtime, often spent enjoying leisure pursuits such as storytelling, cave painting, bead making, or celebrating large kills. Other times would call for an all-out, focused surge that shocked the neuroendocrine (neurotransmitters and hormones) feedback loops—a response to the sudden appearance of, say, a saber-toothed tiger.

Today, our genes still expect occasional short-term shocks, what the scientific community formally refers to as *hormesis*. Of course, these need not be life threatening to be effective. If you have ever jumped into a cold plunge pool and experienced the shock of a sudden drop in temperature, you have experienced hormesis. Not so pleasant, maybe, in the moment, but it feels oh-so-good immediately following. Hence, the popularity of roller coasters and other adrenaline thrills, which we'll cover in the book's last chapter. Such experiences that briefly shock your system provide stimuli for growth. The disconnect here is that many of us find ourselves in long periods of hyperarousal—the classic fight-or-flight response—in our daily lives, which ultimately results in total burnout.

One of the most common ways to pump out some feel-good endorphins is through exercise, something that Grok likely appreciated while running from predators such as that saber-toothed tiger. Instead of tiring out and giving up halfway through the escape, his "runner's high" enabled his brain to signal his legs to keep moving. Of course, we all know exercise makes you feel good and helps you build a strong heart, strong lungs, and strong muscles. But did you know that the proper dose of exercise can also help you build a stronger brain? When you get your blood pumping and muscles working, the neurons in your brain become more flexible and numerous, releasing neurotransmitters such as GABA and dopamine into your bloodstream. These have a calming effect on your nervous system, which in turn helps mitigate the negative effects of stress, anger, anxiety, and depression. Sadly, this potent connection is completely neglected by many of us, ultimately leading to a downward spiral of declining energy and productivity, and leaving us looking in the wrong direction for answers such as ninety-day-crash-fitness courses. Or conversely, in the case of the chronic exerciser, abusing exercise as an addiction to the endorphin high.

THE GENETICS OF CULTURE

We have inherited from our ancestors not just the physical attributes and neural connections that comprise human instinct—such as running from trouble, eating when hungry, or sleeping when tired—but also the capacity to learn and accumulate knowledge, create and appreciate art, socialize, engage in critical thinking and debate, and share these things in a manner that promotes culture and legacy. It was this unique aspect of human evolution that was most influential in our rise to the top of the food chain.

Many of the things that we believe are entirely a product of modern cultural influence actually took genetic root long ago in our species. For example, our elongated childhood and adolescent development has afforded us an intensive period of enculturation for learning the knowledge and practices of the community through play, instruction, and observation. The raucousness and rebellion of the teenage years also serves an evolutionary purpose. It is a necessary (and annoying!) component of an adolescent's transition from a dependent into a confident, self-sustaining adult capable of battling opposing forces and managing life's challenges. Even our penchant for gossip has strong evolutionary roots. Today, gabbing at the water cooler can get us into hot water, but it was exactly this type of chitchat that had once helped clans share and process important social knowledge.

As for our evolutionary history, it began some seven million years ago, when hominids (our prehuman ancestors) split from apes and branched out into various new species. Then, about 2.5 million years ago, the humanlike *Homo erectus* started to take charge of the food chain with their large brains, upright stature, skilled use of tools and fire, and organized hunter-gatherer societies. Over time, *Homo erectus* further branched out into various other hominid subspecies, which included our more immediate ancestors, *Homo sapiens*. British geneticist Stephen Oppenheimer, author of *The Real Eve: Modern Man's Journey Out of Africa* and a leading expert in using DNA to track migration, contends the earliest evidence of our *Homo sapiens* mitochondrial DNA and Y chromosome ancestors came out of East Africa around a hundred and sixty thousand years ago.

For the first one hundred thousand years of *Homo sapiens'* existence, we demonstrated an increasing neurological tendency toward social interaction and the development of language, ritual, trade, art, music, and technology. Most experts believe the final piece of our evolutionary puzzle was a significant genetic mutation that launched us toward modern cognitive and cultural potential, and that this happened around sixty thousand years ago. Richard G. Klein, author of *The Human Career: Human Biological and Cultural Origins*, and others propose that this mutation facilitated a linguistic capacity far more advanced than what hominids had been accustomed to for the previous hundred thousand years.

> **" The development of our cognitively fluid mind amounts to no less than an adaptive home run in the survival-of-the-fittest game. "**

We observe this linguistic phenomenon today in young children, who, across the globe, possess the ability to speak at a comparable and extremely rapid rate, and in similar learning patterns despite highly diverse languages and nurture environments. Noam Chomsky, widely regarded as the father of modern linguistics, asserts grammar—that is, syntax—is the result of a hardwired *language acquisition device* in the human brain, and that all children are born with an inherent aptitude for organizing words into novel sentences. He rejects the idea that children learn grammar by imitating sentences they've heard; rather, their abilities in grammar are innate and coded in our genes. This "universal grammar" trait enables humans to learn any language(s) we are exposed to at a very young age.

Klein believes that this linguistic mutation was "arguably the most important" set of developments in human evolutionary history, for it "produced the fully modern ability to invent and manipulate culture." Not only would such an advance evolve social structure, it would have allowed for, as Klein puts it, more complex "mental modeling," a level of thought and communication that encompassed the pivotal ability to ponder what-if scenarios. Steven Mithen, author of *After the Ice: A Global Human History 20,000–5000 BC*, is among a growing group of anthropologists who believe our species surged ahead when genetic happenstance allowed certain "specialized intelligences" to converge and result in a "cognitively fluid mind."

Experts refer to this convergence as a "symbolic revolution"—a shift that many believe reflects a fully modern cognitive capacity. Consequently, humans started producing significantly more art, ornaments, vessels, and other material goods that suggest a flowering of exchange and social culture unlike that found in previous tool cultures. The real significance of these newer artifacts is their implication of an advanced kinship structure. Archeologist Clive Gamble says the artifacts represent "material metaphors" and "social technologies" that supported kinship as it was to become, stretched across time and space in the expansion of humanity through migration.

The development of our cognitively fluid mind amounts to no less than an adaptive home run in the survival-of-the-fittest game, with, as the widely accepted "out of Africa" theory suggests, an elite group of home-run hitters colonizing the entire globe. Actually, "elite" is an understatement: there were only an estimated two to five thousand humans alive in Africa sixty thousand years ago. We were literally a species on the brink of extinction! And some scientists believe (from studies of carbon-dated cave art, archaeological sites, and human skeletons) that the group that crossed the Red Sea to begin the great migration was a mere one hundred fifty.[8] Only the most innovative survived, carrying with them problem-solving traits that would eventually give rise to our incredible imagination and creativity.

For the first thirty thousand years after leaving Africa, humans endured catastrophic climate changes, which stifled progress. But we ultimately thrived and expanded across the entire continents of Asia and Europe (including Northeast Asia, which poised humans for the eventual migration to the Americas, completed some twelve thousand years ago). In the process, humans prevailed over remaining hominid populations, outliving the Neanderthal in Europe and the *Homo floresiensis* in Asia.

Then, around 28,000 BCE, a dramatic thing started happening: more humans began reaching old age. Professors of anthropology Rachel Caspari of the University of Michigan and Sang-Hee Lee of University of California, Riverside published a 2003 study referencing human fossil records from various time periods. They discovered that molar wear patterns from the Early Upper

Paleolithic period reveal a five-fold increase in the number of individuals surviving to an older age (defined by doubling reproductive age and potentially becoming grandparents). Scientists speculate that the longer life spans hugely contributed to population expansions, cultural innovations, and reinforced family bonds that are now associated with modernity. Elders could pass on critical life knowledge to younger generations, and social networks and family bonds were strengthened. In Caspari's words, the "research provides a simple explanation for which there is now concrete evidence: modern humans were older and wiser."

The evolution of culture by relatively older, wiser, and more creative humans has since predominated over the biological mutations and selections that had defined evolution over the previous couple million years. Culture could now become, as science writer Matt Ridley describes, "progressive [and] cumulative in a way that it simply was not before." Like our need to enjoy nature and music, we humans are hardwired to accumulate and pass along knowledge, but the cultural content that a particular group develops is quite distinct. During primal times, cultural constructs were tied to matters of local survival. If you lived near the ocean, for example, your culture may have centered itself on spearfishing skills. Today, it's a matter of personal preference—finding your calling and realizing your creative, intellectual, and physical potential to make a meaningful contribution to society. As Ridley explains in his book, *The Agile Gene: How Nature Turns on Nurture*, "The difference between me and one of my African ancestors of a hundred thousand years ago is not in our brains or genes, which are basically the same, but in the accumulated knowledge made possible by art, literature, and technology. My brain is stuffed with such information, whereas his larger brain was just as stuffed but with much more local and ephemeral knowledge."

Our advanced cognitive abilities further enhanced our culture, our survival, and—for better or for worse—our inexorable progress in technology. Our genetic predisposition for culture and our insatiable quest for knowledge have represented our greatest strengths as a species, but lately have become the enemy of our health and balance. The hunter-gatherer conditions that prevailed when these traits were selected bear little resemblance to our astoundingly novel modern society. Thanks to technology—and the noise, sound, light, and thought pollution it produces—the fight-or-flight response, our bread and butter throughout evolution, is now one of the most abused mechanisms in the human body.

Our genes have not changed in any significant or health-relevant manner since we transitioned from hunter-gatherer life to civilized life. We are essentially apes with wristwatches and wardrobes. Any desired future updates to your hardwiring are afforded only through tens of thousands of years of life-or-death selection pressure. And those simply aren't going to happen anytime soon. Still, you're free to acquire and expand on the knowledge and experiences of those who walked hundreds, thousands, and millions of years before you, and do so in your own unique way—all within the framework of honoring your primal blueprint. As you get connected, you'll preserve your health, happiness, and, I dare say, sanity.

HAPPINESS VS. PLEASURE

Paradox alert: we are compelled to engage in behaviors that were originally intended to enhance survival, but do so in a world where there is no selection pressure! Hence, we can and do hijack these ancient biochemical reward pathways with all sorts of instant gratifications and addictive behaviors. Witness the junkie in the street, the chronic overeater, or even Tiger Woods and his adulterous frolicking, driven by primordial forces that, back in the day, helped ensure the hardy existence of our species. Such behavior today, however, conflicts with established social constructs and mores, and for Tiger, it cost him his family and hundreds of million of dollars in endorsements.

The simple answer, one that Grok likely understood but we often need to be reminded of, is to balance our urges with common sense. Tap into your genetic ability to ponder what-if scenarios, and use the system for its intended purpose: to guide you toward smart choices that benefit your long-term health, happiness, and wellness. I think we can all imagine the decision Grok would have made had he been faced with a cause-and-effect scenario, say discovering an inviting watering hole to cool off in but also finding that it fronts a den of saber-toothed tigers!

Remember, too, that Grok's world was largely one of scarcity. There was a real adaptive benefit for hormonal and neurochemical reinforcements in such a world, where coming across a beehive filled with honey was like finding gold. Even fruit was quite a prize, though often less sweet than tart. The disconnect today is overabundance and easy access to these once-rare inputs. We now can, at will, self-stimulate our innate reward system. Go by any store, and you are greeted with a rack of candy out front. The hardwiring that has reinforced our survival for millions of years has now potentially become, if we do not honor it properly, our biggest enemy.

Some tied to the modern ideas of psychology might call this invoking our higher cognitive powers—what Freud famously labeled the ego and the super-ego—weighing the short-term payoffs of our actions against the long-term consequences. I prefer to just say: take responsibility for your actions as you seek pleasure.

And seek pleasure you must. You owe it to your genes. There is a biochemical reason that dirt makes you happy, why providing for your family gives you a sense of accomplishment and security, and why puttering in your garden or garage workshop can generate more satisfaction at the biochemical level than closing yet another million-dollar business deal or winning another important golf tournament. A funny movie, throwing the Frisbee with your dog at the park, eating a basket of fresh cherries, or taking a soak in the tub all ignite your internal reward system and deliver instant pleasure. Make such indulgences a regular feature in your life, not just a few fleeting moments grasped here and there. When we make healthful, simple pleasures a priority, we are rewarded with a lifetime of happiness. Believe me, we humans are really good at this—it's hardwired in our genes!

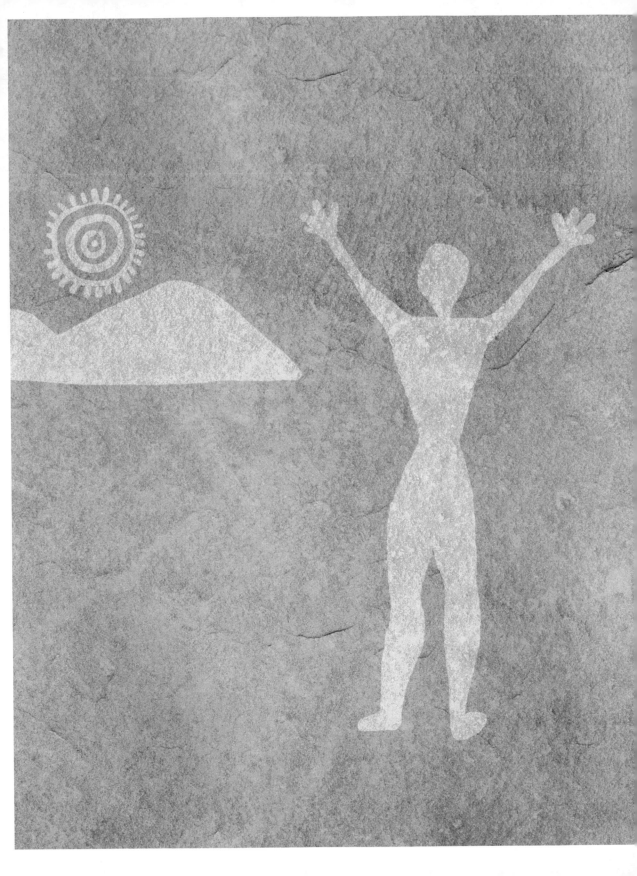

THE INNER DIALOGUE CONNECTION

WHETHER IT IS THE PERCEPTION of our successes or failures, or whether it is our self-judgment or guilt or depression—our self-chatter gets in our way. Such is the destruction of negative self-talk, an artifact of language. We're blessed with so much. We should be happy. Yet we analyze and relive past interactions, we emotionally narrate our experiences, we obsess about superficial concerns, worry over the imagined outcome of events. Then there are all the questions: what's broken? What is it that is not working, not consistent, not resonating? Why can't I get more done? When am I ever going to have time for all the things—the goals, the plans, the people I've been putting off? We wonder if there is something more. Except maybe it's not about more…. Maybe it's about relearning our old ancestral habits.

Attitude is a little thing that makes a big difference.

WINSTON CHURCHILL

THE INNER DIALOGUE CONNECTION

BEFORE WE GO ANY FURTHER, let's pull back for some perspective. It's important to step out of our modern mindset and think more like a hunter-gatherer. It's really not that much of a stretch. It's still there, still part of who we are if we're willing to accept it—and access it. When we bring a primal perspective to our lives, we can begin to make key connections. We can begin to see our choices differently.

Let's start with our inner chatter. We spend a lot of time in our heads these days. We mentally catalogue our to-do lists and check off logistical notes throughout the day. We emotionally narrate our experiences, respond to what is said and not said, analyze every nuance of our conversations, and even relive past interactions, often judging or beating ourselves up in the process. Then there are the big questions of ongoing self-talk we use to define ourselves. It's interesting that we put such a substantial premium on "finding ourselves." We use this phrase to suggest an essential quest or—in the absence of knowing—a crisis. We ask, "Who am I?" "What is my life about?" "What should it be about?" "What makes for a happy, fulfilled, balanced life?"

As common as the questions are, satisfactory answers all too often elude us. In the end, most of our self-chatter leads us to feel lost, discontented, even

THE 10 HABITS OF HIGHLY SUCCESSFUL HUNTER-GATHERERS

 Take responsibility

 Be selfish

 Build a tribe

 Be present

 Be curious

 Trust your gut

 Pick your battles

 Get over it

 Sharpen your spear

 Be affluent

defeated. For all our self-analysis, why do we seem to be more confused about who we are and less satisfied with what we have than previous generations?

The problem is we overthink, we overreact, we self-criticize, and we self-judge … because we can. That's the irony. We get bound into distorting our own realities. We cut ourselves off from what's essential. Tens of thousands of years ago, we evolved some pretty elaborate cognitive abilities like self-awareness and metarepresentation. And with those gifts, we learned to process what-if scenarios and grasp the emotional complexity of—and separateness between—ourselves and others. The adaptive benefits of these developments included being able to assess our own motives and imagine those of others—for example, reasoning that your buddy will probably be upset if you strike up a relationship with his lady friend. And mulling over all kinds of hypotheticals in selecting the best course of action such as deducing that it is probably safer to kill a mammoth with a projectile spear rather than to run up on it and jab it with your stone-carved knife.

Though beneficial much of the time, these cognitive abilities can become intellectual and emotional traps when they aren't brought into check by the social environment that first defined them. Our brains formed in a simpler time and environment. It was pretty clear what was real and what wasn't; and what wasn't real was inconsequential. Today, we make what isn't real our reality. We literally dream up ways to make our lives more difficult and miserable. We spend hours obsessing in front of mirrors when our ancient ancestors never in their lives saw a full image of their own reflection. We compare ourselves to digitally enhanced people on magazine covers, who in reality have no connection to our lives. We secretly eye the count of Facebook friends of people we know, convinced our own social circles must be lacking. We relive the anguish of past insults, refusing to acknowledge that the events are done, and hence current pains are self-initiated. We worry needlessly over possible future events that exist for now only in our thoughts, and yet they cause us to back off or shut down. In going down these imaginary roads, we entertain thoughts of ingratitude, resentment, self-doubt, depression, and, in some cases, even suicide.

Once upon a time, self-reflection served a valuable purpose that was rooted in the stakes of survival. Today, it more often just gets in the way of authentic living with relentless self-chatter that distorts our own sense of wellbeing. It ultimately diminishes the experience of the present moment, and keeps us from giving our focus and energy to what can genuinely serve our health and fulfillment.

In fact, we can get stuck in self-talk as a confining, even sabotaging condition. When we follow the path of self-talk to its logical (or illogical) conclusion, we often act completely against our self-interest. Consider the concept of akrasia. It encompasses this irrational, confounding state of mind in which we wittingly throw caution, reason, and consequences to the wind in order to pursue a choice we know will be bad for us.

> ❝ **Survival required that our ancestors regroup and forge ahead to the next challenge when they faced unfavorable circumstances.** ❞

Examples of akrasia include dumping your healthful diet for an emotionally charged binge with a quart of chocolate ice cream. And then indulging in the guilt afterwards. Or in procrastinating on something important, such as putting off working on your tax return until the second week in April, or avoiding cleaning out the refrigerator until you'd rather throw out the Tupperware than open the lid.

We get it intellectually, but something illusory and emotional takes over. Strictly speaking, we know better. In fact, we know pretty much exactly what repercussions will befall us—financial trouble, relationships fallouts, job stress, health effects, and so on—but damned if we don't go down that road anyway.

Some just shrug their shoulders and suggest it is simply human nature. Can we truly write off our responsibility so easily as chalking it up to "hominids will be hominids?" As much as we're subject to evolutionary instincts, we generally have enough thinking skills on the higher order to pull ourselves back from the brink when we're so inclined.

The fact is, we're all subject to the conflicting impulses and better spirits of our human heritage. When we each consider what has caused us to act against our self-interest, what has held us back from embracing better choices at certain points in our lives, rarely does it ever come down to any neat, academic abstraction. Instead, it's a long, intricate yarn of personal experience.

Part of self-control is self-understanding: knowing the circumstances that test your confidence, preempting the script that tends to play in your head when life gets tough or you have time on your hands. Only then can you divert the narrative, anticipate your needs, and genuinely tend to your weaknesses before they get the better of you. It's about understanding that this, too, shall pass. The power to consciously steer your own self-talk today determines who, and what, ultimately directs your overall life story.

How, then, do we rein in this penchant for the self-talk that undermines genuine and healthy self-interest? How do we impose perspective and proportion on what ultimately matters? Try putting the focus of your self-talk against the backdrop of our Paleolithic ancestors, and see what it looks like. Chances are, the vast majority of your inner chatter will appear pretty inconsequential. When we reconnect with our fundamental roots and follow those habits, we are better able to assess what's real and healthy and what's just mentally contrived nonsense. We are able to cultivate a more balanced, focused, and stable sense of self. We are better able to fully appreciate the adage: *Life is 10 percent what happens to us* (chance) *and 90 percent how we respond to it* (choice).

In making the Primal Connection, there are inevitably layers of modern clutter and distortion to shuck. The process obliges us to release ingrained behaviors—like our inner dialogue—that hinder opportunities for pleasure, happiness, and fulfillment. We need to recognize these obstructions, recalibrate our lives, and restore equilibrium. Consider the journey a homecoming to the natural default point, a center from which we can re-engage the genuine rewards of living the full measure of our essential humanity. Now let's take a look at the 10 Habits of Highly Successful Hunter-Gatherers. Think of them as a set of tools that will give you an evolutionary perspective and help you navigate the rest of this book.

TAKE RESPONSIBILITY

Perhaps the most powerful and uniquely human trait of our hunter-gatherer ancestors was their full acknowledgment of life's realities as well as its cruelties. If you can tap into this one part of the Primal Connection fully, every other piece of information will seem to fall into place effortlessly. I assure you, it isn't an easy fix, as we have been socialized to blame our predicament on anything and everyone but ourselves, but it is essential to achieving peace and balance.

Nowadays we have the luxury of wallowing in despair, self-pity, self-judgment, or doubt. Not so in Grok's day. Life was harsh, unforgiving, and unrelenting in throwing challenges at our hunter-gatherer ancestors. Can you imagine them moping around with their heads hung low, judging themselves as failures when they didn't catch the beast they had been tracking, or when they discovered that the water source they'd finally found was tainted? Highly unlikely! Maybe disappointed, but to the hunter-gatherer, a victim mindset would have been a sure recipe for death. As Art DeVany, author of *The New Evolution Diet*, is fond of saying, to the hunter-gatherer, there is no failure—only feedback. Indeed, survival required that our ancestors regroup and forge ahead to the next challenge when they faced unfavorable circumstances. Sure, our ancestors did things with a purpose (a goal), but had the outcome not been to their advantage, they likely accepted it and moved on, trying again later or devising an alternate plan.

This is what owning your life, owning your problems, and owning the outcome looked like ten thousand years ago. This is what taking responsibility for your life—everything that has ever happened to you, and everything that ever will happen to you—should look like today. Picture the modern human wearing a suit instead of animal skins and hunting for a job instead of a beast. Same genetic recipe and proclivities, simply a different set of circumstances.

Taking responsibility for your life doesn't mean that you have to lay blame on yourself. What I'm talking about here is choice, and how you choose to respond to any given situation. It could be that you had a spate of bad luck, were born into less-than-ideal circumstances, had abusive parents, fell in with the wrong crowd, or just got bad information. It means that you don't make excuses, and you don't necessarily place blame on others for your current sour situation. Hey, it could technically be someone else's "fault," but blaming allows you to languish in the presumed comfort of bad habits. It allows you to stew in self-pity, to accept inertia for the sake of ongoing bitterness. Yet, blame always betrays you in the end. Whatever excuses you tell yourself day after day, the sense of loss—of being locked outside of your own life—is still there. It's a grief that leaves you hollowed out and estranged. Responsibility is your

YOU ARE HARDWIRED *to respond as well as react.*

MODERN DISCONNECT: *reacting to situations that require a thoughtful response.*

PRIMAL CONNECTION: *give up the blame game and take responsibility.*

acceptance of the situation, your acknowledgment that however it happened, you are the only one who can make the choices to get yourself out.

Unlike other animals, humans evolved an ability to *respond* emotionally to situations, rather than simply to *react* rationally. Reaction is the province of the fight-or-flight system that predates humans by hundreds of millions of years. Reaction is wired into our reptilian brains as a survival mechanism. It doesn't require much thought; it's automatic. On the other hand, the brain's neocortex (evolved over millions of years with aid of our high-fat diet) can override the knee-jerk, fight-or-flight reactions typical of most other species and run quickly through various what-if scenarios and plot alternative strategies for myriad life-threatening encounters.

Nevertheless, despite our ability to think our way out of a tight spot, our fight-or-flight tendencies are deeply rooted . The skill to separate, or appropriately integrate, our two modes of thinking (react blindly or respond intelligently—we call it "response ability") can make a huge difference in your own life, whether it has to do with finances, health, relationships, or real survival situations.

Like our ancestors, every morning we wake up to face a day of uncertainty. Recognize that bad things happen all the time. But how we deal with those things is ours and ours alone. If you get rear-ended at a stoplight, it may not be your fault, but the choices you made put you in that place, on that day, and at that time. Acknowledge and accept the problem, and consider your available choices—including whether or not you will allow this to ruin your day or week.

If you are addicted to pain pills, in an unhappy marriage, struggling with your weight, or one of the millions on their way to type 2 diabetes, be brutally honest with yourself right now, and ask what behaviors, actions, and decisions you made to be in the situation you are in currently. If there is even the remotest hint of excuse or blame, you are not in control of your own destiny. You are essentially allowing life to happen, like a boat lost at sea without a captain.

In finally giving up the blame game, we make peace with the complexity and difficulty of life. We shake off the last of our excuses, and let go of the martyr role. We become the essence of the hunter-gatherer. True, life isn't always fair. We don't get to choose every circumstance. We don't get to control the people around us. Likewise, we don't get all the time in the world to wait for the ideal circumstances to come around. Life, as we all eventually come to understand (hopefully before it's too late), will never be perfect. There will always be obstacles, annoyances, and limitations to contend with on our paths. Regardless of what your life looks like next to someone else's, yours is still the one you go home with at the end of the day. Yours is the one you get to live—for all its possibility as well as challenge. The question is: what will you make of it today?

FEED THE HABIT:

Think about your own life right now. How would you describe your health? Your overall sense of wellbeing? What have been your challenges? What have been the high points of your life? Where do you feel limited? How do you feel supported? What gives you strength and joy? What do you long for? The point here is to understand the story and intentions that you bring to your life's journey. Look at the following list of concepts and relate them to your life right now. Acknowledge the first words that come to mind as you read each.

Vitality	Satisfaction	Community
Composure	Vigor	Exuberance
Pleasure	Intimacy	Creativity
Intention	Progress	Spirit
Rest	Contentment	Balance
Abundance	Leisure	

Now think about these same concepts again, only this time in relation to your desired life. Ask yourself this: what is standing in the way of achieving this life? What are the obstacles that block your path? Specific circumstances? Lack of energy? Lack of time? Lack of direction? Stress? Illness? Anger? Emptiness? Misguided priorities? Entrenched habit? Now evaluate your choices. Begin steering your life with those that best align with your desired destination.

Set up a WTF Fund. Stuff happens in life, and sometimes it costs money to fix. No reason to get upset. Create a separate budgetary item made up of spare change, $20 a week, or a small percentage of your paycheck. When a WTF moment happens—a broken window, overpaying for a good or service, or seeing a family member buy something you deem as irresponsible or excessive—don't be a victim. Tap into your WTF Fund and fugetaboutit!

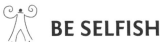 **BE SELFISH**

What kind of entity is it that survives, or does not survive, as a consequence of natural selection? This is the question Richard Dawkins asked as he penned his seminal work *The Selfish Gene*. He later lamented that he should have titled the book *The Immortal Gene* or even *The Altruistic Vehicle*, because in reality his book detailed how altruism figured greatly in the evolution of our species. In order to survive, we fed and protected our kin who shared copies of our genetic material. We evolved depending on and cooperating with the small group to which we were attached, always recognizing that survival is nearly impossible without the support of others. We indeed had serious motivation to get along, to pitch in, to be, well, altruistic. Yet the human race could not have survived without a degree of selfishness. After all, the caveman ethos is not that of a martyr.

Being selfish does not mean valuing yourself above all others. It means being as generous with yourself as you are with others. If you believe that all people should be protected, nurtured, loved, and filled with joy, then recognize that you are a person, too, deserving of all those things as well. No one is better equipped to provide that to you than yourself. For example, consider the go-to person at the office, the one everyone can count on to put in the extra hours and get the work done. He has a hard time saying no, and maybe a part of him secretly enjoys carrying the extra burden. But under the crush of trying to please and taking on too much, it is often at the expense of his physical, emotional, and mental health. Ultimately, unless he pays attention to this, he will burn out. We see intimate relationships undergo a similar fate when one lover assigns a disproportionate amount of time and energy to the other. The latter eventually feels stifled while the former feels resentful. How might these scenarios play out differently if the selfless became a little more considerate of their own wellbeing—negotiating for more time on a project or additional help, or investing time and energy in self-improvement rather than slavishly doting on another who may or may not appreciate it?

Essentially, it all boils to down how you determine your decisions. Start by consulting yourself first. How do you feel about the issue? How does it supply your needs or infringe upon them? What do you want? Once you have a baseline of your own position, then and only then do you expand the question to that of anyone else involved, or affected. You may opt to consider others over yourself in the end, but you will have done so with a clear and compelling reason to acquiesce to other purposes. You will have made a choice, and choices are what it's all about.

Of course, parenting, by definition, is a selfless endeavor in which we choose to participate. We enter the parenting game knowing this, and the rewards we reap in return are immeasurable. But when self-sacrifice is taken to the extreme, when you are beginning to indulge the *wants* of your children before your own basic *needs*, it may be time to pull back and re-evaluate. I'm talking about running yourself ragged working a second job so that you can earn the money to buy your children new video games and designer clothes, yet you haven't any spare time to spend with your children, let alone get enough sleep. I'm talking about not setting boundaries, the inability to say no, and doing things for your children that they could do themselves such as cleaning their rooms instead of assigning chores. At the end of the day, the question then becomes what sort of role model do you want to be for your children to emulate once they grow up and become parents themselves?

Think of it this way: the more you sacrifice your own health, happiness, and sanity, the less you have to give. Conversely, when you have a healthy relationship with yourself, the happier and better off you are, and therefore the more valuable your gifts to others will become. You become a better lover, a better parent, a better volunteer, a better employee, a better member of society. Simply put, we have to help ourselves before we can help others. We are reminded of this simple principle every time we board a plane and are instructed to put on our own oxygen mask first before assisting our family members in the event of an emergency. The truth is, we simply cannot be altruistic without being selfish first. Just don't go overboard and sacrifice other people's welfare in pursuit of your own.

FEED THE HABIT:

Treat yourself to some guilt-free me-time. Carve out some time and spend a day at the spa, take a drive up the coast, relish a lazy day on the couch reading a novel, enjoy a long soak in the tub, or play golf in the middle of the week.

YOU ARE HARDWIRED *for altruism as well as personal survival.*

MODERN DISCONNECT: *playing the martyr.*

PRIMAL CONNECTION: *love and take care of yourself first.*

Find an old picture of yourself, one of you as a child. What would you like to do for that child? What does that child need that you can give him or her now? If it's a trip to the zoo, go. If it's more complicated (and whose life isn't?) list out the challenges, and write about what thoughts or actions you would need to better nurture your inner child.

Have kinder communications with yourself. Instead of negative self-talk, try saying positive words like *joy, love, life, happy, strong, beautiful, tranquility.* Affirmations are wonderfully healing, too, especially those starting with the words, *I am. I am healthy. I am happy. I am positive.*

BUILD A TRIBE

A strong social circle for our hunter-gatherer forebears was a given. As we've just learned, in the harsh circumstances of their time, it would've been near impossible to scratch out a life alone. Instead, they lived within the security of a band community—a kinship group of approximately twenty-five to seventy people. Some within the group were related. Others were not. Participation within the group was more than simple transaction or familial affiliation. Kinship was created through a sense of mutuality—forged in action. The bond was born out of continual, concrete participation in the group—in engaging with the hunting and foraging that would feed the community; in protecting the group from predators or in the occasional skirmish with another band; in aiding the group with building shelters, creating vessels and weapons, or caring for children; in sharing celebrations; and in receiving the group's aid and support.

What a contrast to think that these days people can go through their adult lives with few, if any, intimate connections. It isn't that we've outgrown the need for kinship. We still, after all, have the same genes that promoted social connection for the sake of survival hundreds of thousands of years ago. What's changed is our culture. We no longer necessarily stay in our hometowns or even home countries. We may live thousands of miles away from our families of origin and childhood friends. In fact, we may make several geographical relocations in our lives for school, work, marriage, or whim. Even if we stay in one place for a long stretch, we get busy, life gets complicated, and we lose touch. As a result, many of us end up feeling unattached, socially adrift.

Wherever and at whatever time in your life you find yourself now, it's imperative to build a tribe. The irony of doing so in this day and age, of course, is we live every day in proximity to thousands of people as opposed to the few and far between as our ancestors did. We have hundreds of social media connections but few real relationships. The truth is, exposure doesn't fill our social wells. It's about solid, mutually supportive relationships. A tribe here represents people with whom you feel closest, the people you feel know you the best and have seen you through life transitions or meaningful events. Likewise, you've done the same for them. You have a history, and likely a lot of stories that can keep you reminiscing deep into the night. These relationships include your life partner, your kids, your family of origin, and maybe closer members of your extended family. But it's also—and for some people more so—intimate friends. These are the friends you can drop by and visit unannounced. They're the ones you can call—and call upon—at all hours.

Bottom line, if you don't have a family, make one. If you don't have a core group, build one. Don't tell yourself you missed the boat on this one. Don't tell yourself you're too busy. This is too important.

Sure, making friends as an adult isn't the casual, happenstance arrangement that it is when you're a kid or even when you're in college, but it's just as vital and rewarding. Sociology professor Rebecca G. Adams from the University of Carolina at Greensboro explains the three keys that are essential to form intimate friendships: "proximity; repeated, unplanned interactions; and a setting that encourages people to let their guard down and confide in each other."[1] Ask yourself what kind of people you want to be surrounded by, and ask yourself what you have to offer in return. Go to the places where they go. Introduce yourself. Participate. Initiate connections.

This said, bring a genuine interest in the people you encounter. Ask questions and make eye contact. And don't limit yourself to finding your personal doppelgänger. Conversations with people who hold a different point of view from yours can make for lively conversation. Prioritize key principles, but bring an otherwise open attitude. Offer trustworthiness and respect as well as pragmatism. If they don't return the same level of interest, move on rather than waste your time and emotional investment. Along that vein, think quality over quantity. Cultivate the relationships you think you have the time, motivation, and energy to maintain. A few genuine friendships are more rewarding than a hundred acquaintances.

FEED THE HABIT:

Foster relationships within the connections you already have. There's no need to start from scratch. Think of people you already know but with whom you never had the chance to develop something more involved, or reconnect with old acquaintances through an alumni group. Put yourself out there and extend a personal invitation.

Lead with your personal interests. Take a class. Join a sports league, running club, book group, or professional organization. Try a Meetup group in your area. You won't only be meeting like-minded people, but you'll have the ongoing chance to build a relationship over time. And—if nothing else—you'll enjoy the activity just for its own sake.

Be an organizer. Take the bull by the horns and throw a party. Coordinate a volunteer team at work. Start a fantasy sports league or mothers' group. You'd be surprised how many people want to connect as much as you do but are just as intimidated by getting the ball rolling.

Bring your best to the relationship and look for the same. You're looking for people who can be positive, enriching, supportive friends. Offer that in return. Even long-term friendships can go south if one person constantly unloads or if the routine becomes too ho-hum. Renew the energy and interest in your friendships—new and old.

 # BE PRESENT

For our hunter-gatherer ancestors, life was an exercise in hypervigilance. Life in the wild allowed for very little leeway in awareness. Picture a hunter-gatherer examining subtle patterns of broken twigs and bent grasses as he tracked prey. At turns, he would stop to smell the breeze and seek out whiffs of scat. He lived life in the imperative of the now. Though he and his kind lived lives consisting of large amounts of downtime, they were rarely afforded the luxury of "checking out" mentally, lest they become the prey instead of the predator. It wasn't just the business of hunting—or avoiding being hunted—either. Attentiveness mattered to all of life and livelihood then. Our hunter-gatherer forebears deciphered sensory cues that signaled migratory patterns, edible plants, water sources, navigation cues, impending weather, and the occasional outsiders' presence. Distraction could mean missing essential clues that would make the difference between a healthy meal and a deadly one, a route to resource-rich land and a path to nowhere. Being present meant not getting lost on the way home. It meant staying alive.

By contrast, we moderns are used to walking through life preoccupied. You see it everywhere—people absorbed in their phones as they walk down the street, or as they stave off their young children's efforts for attention. There's always some harried businessman rushing through pedestrian traffic muttering a frustrated obscenity under his breath.

Whether it's technology or mental chatter, we're chronically lost in distractions of our own making. We justify it as multitasking, except each task suffers with every additional undertaking. It's about letting constant distraction hijack the full experience of life. How often are we preoccupied by everything but the people, places, and possibilities right in front of us? Our enslavement to diversion suggests a strangling self-absorption. In our ancestors' day, it would've been our fatal undoing. Today, it's "merely" a psychological burden we continually impose on our psyches. We're locked inside ourselves, more often than not, disconnected from the world and people around us.

In terms of business, our diverted attentions sacrifice efficiency and creativity. As research demonstrates, multitasking doesn't save us time and brainpower. Our learning capacity actually diminishes when we multitask, taxing our short-term memory unnecessarily. Furthermore, we miss out on the creative and emotional benefits of flow, that state of mind in which self-consciousness slips away in a larger, engrossing challenge. In these hyperfocused moments, we experience the rewards of emotional release as well as creative productivity, much the way our ancestors did during their daily endeavors.

YOU ARE HARDWIRED *for single-minded focus.*

MODERN DISCONNECT: *rampant distraction.*

PRIMAL CONNECTION: *give the moment full attention.*

When it comes to our relationships, distraction means we forgo the intimacy that builds genuine connection. Too often we skate over the surface of relating, always caught in one more thought, one more email, one more list. We'll focus after just this "one last thing," we say, but somehow there's always another task, message, or diversion waiting. Your kids and partners, friends and relatives all sense when you're distracted. Imagine giving them your full sensory, intellectual, and emotional presence. Can you remember what that feels like? Can they? Make the commitment to be fully present for them. Let yourself be taken in by their smiles, their conversation, their closeness. Being in the moment with someone means giving that person your whole self as well as your full attention. Your loved ones deserve nothing less.

FEED THE HABIT:

Observe your loved ones. Watch your children play. Listen to their voices and laughter. Look them in the eyes when you speak with them. Absorb the subtle changes in their growing selves. Embed in your mind the memory of your partner's laughter or an aging parent's mannerisms. The people you love change every day. Don't miss it.

Identify twenty things you haven't noticed before. Next time you take a walk through your neighborhood or a familiar natural environment, act like a hunter-gatherer and catalogue your surroundings. Make it a habit each time you venture out for a walk.

Take up a meditative practice. Research demonstrates that meditation, yoga, Tai Chi, and visualization improves attention skills. They can also help quiet the "monkey mind," a yoga term for that unrelenting, manic, mental busyness that won't let you slow down and empty your thoughts.

Incorporate mindfulness check-ins throughout your day. Whether or not you meditate each day, resolve to infuse your life with a more mindful presence. Regular check-ins throughout the day—at breakfast with your spouse, on your lunch hour walk, during quality time with your kids—help you improve mindfulness as a way of living.

BE CURIOUS

As children we have an eager, spastic attraction to the new, the mysterious, the out of reach. From that infinite string of "why" questions to the unrelenting energy for the day's adventures, curiosity is a near constant impulse. Life is to be probed, painted, taken apart, reconstructed, and fit into a fantasy tale with action figures. We tend to interpret these memories as the nostalgic stuff of childhood—adventures in naïveté in the early throes of encountering our small worlds. Ah, but it is so much more. Engaging our curiosity is a universal, adaptive human impulse—one that should be encouraged throughout life.

Humans didn't evolve a particularly imposing size, defensive shell, or threatening physical features. We developed wits instead. In a dicey survival situation, our ancestors depended on knowledge and creative ability to manipulate their physical environments or predatory opponents. They learned to use all manner of natural materials to create shelter, devise medicinal treatment, and incorporate nutritional fortification, through observation and imagination.

We moderns are products of our ancestors' genetically programmed curiosity. When we think of the older people we know who seem the most youthful and fascinating, they're undoubtedly the ones who never stopped exploring, discovering, learning. They are always reading several books. They travel. They start their own business or adopt a second vocation late in life. They love sampling new recipes or visiting the latest restaurants in town. They attend lectures and cultural events. They are always building something. For them, life is an adventure, no matter how many years they have left to explore. They remind us that there is always something fortifying to the pursuit, the question, the revelation.

Life is an open invitation to discover. It's a question of how we engage with our world, how we apprehend and encounter the stimuli around us. Do we go through life with senses turned off, suspended in the thoughts of the next task, or do we bring presence, openness, and curiosity? It's worth asking, how often do you seek out novelty of any kind? Do you feel—and follow—curiosity? When was the last time you felt like you really learned something or have grown

YOU ARE HARDWIRED *for curiosity.*

MODERN DISCONNECT: *ennui, burnout, resting on our laurels.*

PRIMAL CONNECTION: *push your boundaries and try new things.*

from something? We have the potential to challenge our limits and learning throughout the full span of our lives—if we choose to.

FEED THE HABIT:

Be a lifelong learner and commit to a continual education. Read widely and deeply. Watch documentaries. Take classes. Attend seminars. Volunteer. Travel when time and money allow. One educational travel resource to check out is RoadScholar.org. For brain games that will enhance your memory, attention, and creativity look into Lumosity.com.

Connect with others who want to learn and question. There's nothing as inspiring as a long, rousing conversation late into the night about the deep subjects of life. Have people in your life (ideally not of the same opinions) with whom you can share this experience.

Push your personal boundaries. Try new activities on a monthly if not weekly basis. Try a cultural cuisine you've never eaten. Visit a new museum. Take in a play, concert, or sporting event that's unlike anything you've attended before.

Explore new hobbies. Don't just read about new subjects, *do them*. Take up woodworking, weaving, clock building, pottery, gardening, or carpentry. Learn how to sew your own clothes or make your own masterpiece recipes. Fix your own car or build your own backyard shed. There's little to nothing you can't learn if you commit yourself to the endeavor.

 # TRUST YOUR GUT

An extraordinary confluence of sensory abilities helped our ancestors survive a complex, dangerous, and unpredictable world. Acute hearing warned them of approaching predators. A sensitive sense of smell allowed them to anticipate weather and track prey. Sharp and discerning sight helped them differentiate between edible and inedible plants, and navigate both land and open water. Although predominantly a blend of intense sensory awareness, this perceptiveness also incorporated intuitive discernment, a rapid-reasoning neural network that was by itself critically adaptive.

We observe how animals act upon what we call intuition. They seek shelter from storms and natural disasters before people pick up any detectable signs. It's likely that humans at one time had all the same intuitive abilities as our animal cohorts. The fact is, even traditional hunter-gatherer groups today show perception so keen that it can smack of mysticism. Experts are somewhat split on whether we still retain the full measure of these capacities. However, research involving traditional societies and laboratory observation suggests that we still possess key intuitive abilities—and that they play a crucial role in our everyday existence.[2]

We feel intuition viscerally because it's very much a bodily perception. It's a nonverbal, untraceable insight that is actually assembled from perceptual cues, emotional associations, past physical experience, and genetically programmed instincts—often within a split-second. In that way, intuition can seem like an animalistic force, what anthropologist Robert Wolff calls an ancient way of knowing.[3] Although decidedly primal, intuition is hardly an obsolete mode of processing. Even in the twenty-first century, we remain creatures of "dual processing," the intuitive and the intellectual. The key is giving each their proper due.

Experts have long searched for the "seat" of intuition. It's more likely to be part of a complex network than a lone site in our physiological makeup. From a sensory angle, we respond to visual input too fleeting to consciously register. We pick up on everything from subtle facial expressions to hormonal secretions in sizing up or just living with another person. In a fraction of a second, information gets routed through a map of neurological shortcuts—within and outside the actual brain. Before your higher-order thinking can even begin to kick in, the "second brain" of your enteric nervous system (yes, truly your gut) is already giving you feedback. That bad feeling in the pit of your stomach is a legitimate message created in the larger network of neurohormonal production and communication.

YOU ARE HARDWIRED *to be intuitive.*

MODERN DISCONNECT: *overthinking problems and second-guessing solutions.*

PRIMAL CONNECTION: *trust your gut.*

We humans have evolved amazing abilities of higher cognition, but we pay a price for that as well. Although our intuitive powers have likely diminished compared to that of other mammals, we—much to our detriment—tend to discount our intuition wholesale.

How many times have you made a decision in life and immediately descended into a cascade of second-guessing because your neocortex was late in the game with its logical what-if scenarios? Maybe you've experienced changing your mind based on this rationalist rebellion only to later regret the switch after you see the undesirable result. If only I'd gone with my gut, you think.

Research confirms that we often make better decisions—and are more satisfied with our choices—when we rely on intuition rather than reasoning.[4] For instance, we tend to think our conscious mind makes fairer judgments,

> **“ Traditional hunter-gatherer groups today show perception so keen that it can smack of mysticism. ”**

but research suggests we're perhaps more beholden to biases in the decisions we make with conscious deliberation. And we think less creatively when we rely on conscious thought. The subconscious mind, not surprisingly, is better than the conscious one at thinking "out of the box." In a series of studies, the best solutions and choices were made by those who were given a question and then distracted for a short period of time, rather than given time to consciously reflect on the decision, or asked to answer right away.[5] Anyone frustrated by a problem who has found an answer after getting up and walking around the block has experienced this phenomenon. Absolutely, conscious deliberation allows us to work collectively, engage willpower, and shift habits. Your higher brain, for example, is much more likely to resist that bag of M&M's next to you at the checkout. Nonetheless, there's more truth and innovation to be had in the full integration of your cognitive, human self. You'll find genuine guidance when you trust your gut.

FEED THE HABIT:
Get in touch with your own decision-making center. Recognize the conscious "voices" in your decision making—the psychological baggage of bad experiences and misguided authority figures. Clear out the emotional clutter of the past that keeps creeping into your life choices.

When you need to make a decision or approach a problem creatively, stop mulling and step away from the issue. Give yourself a break with some other activity and let your subconscious mind take a stab at it. Head out for a run, take the night to socialize, or try one of the above ideas to mute the rationalist volume and give your subconscious some air space.

PICK YOUR BATTLES

For our hunter-gatherer forebears, life was an exercise in cost-benefit analysis. Did it pay to migrate during a certain season? Was it worth the risk to try hunting bigger predators? How did the time collecting and preparing a certain plant for eating stack up against the taste and satiation? Unless there was something substantial to be gained that made the endeavor worth the extra effort, danger, or conflict, our ancestors favored choices that conserved their energy, minimized risk, and maintained band equilibrium.

Despite our lives of unprecedented choice and ease, we'd still do well to apply the same principle: lead with the priorities. There are the practical choices. By way of illustration, is it worth paying someone twice the amount to drywall the basement when you could probably do a decent job yourself with a bigger time investment? It's a call you base on how much or how little free time you have versus spare cash.

Beyond these literal cost-benefit equations, however, exist the more emotional and social considerations you make every day. How do you invest your time and energy in your relationships? How much of your engagement goes to doling out orders and criticism—however "constructive" you believe them to be? What else could—or should—you be seeing and appreciating in others if you let more of the negatives slide?

In a situation that would normally ruffle your feathers, ask yourself what you stand to gain by fighting the battle. Is this battle substantial or essential? Does the situation even require your response? To every action, there's an opposite reaction. Consider what and who you will be upsetting if you go down this road. Perhaps there could be ramifications. Think about what you may bring down on yourself with this battle, maybe losing a client, alienating your partner, or disappointing your children.

Choosing an unnecessary battle won't unravel your life in one bout. However, if you can't back away from constant criticism or refuse to let go of anything, you can gradually wear away and close off the intimacy and good will of your relationships—from business connections to intimate partnerships. Moreover, continually engaging in cynicism has a tendency to just plain wear you down.

At a certain point, constant battles suggest an inability to compromise. It implies an inability to respect the full humanity of other people and the unpredictable nature of life itself. A will to control wouldn't have been tolerated in the autonomy-minded hunter-gatherer culture. Today, you might not literally be voted off the island as you perhaps would've been then, but you'll eventually make yourself irrelevant and unwelcome.

The larger lesson runs deeper than simply cutting back on negativity, however. It obliges us to think about how we approach our relationships and how our own sense of self enriches or impairs our connections. Maybe you haven't identified what the core priorities are in your life yet. That's critical personal work. The longer you put it off, the more conflict and lost opportunity you'll undoubtedly bring upon yourself. There's no single or fixed answer, but it's a question that engages your expectations of life and other people, as well as your own self-knowledge and healthy sense of humility. People in old age often share how the end of life brings perspective to what really matters. Impending loss is perhaps the ultimate lens on such things. Nonetheless, our experience and reflection throughout our lives teach us, if we let them.

Finally, we can choose our battles wisely when it comes to our own self-development. Selecting your most valued goals and releasing others isn't an exercise in defeat. Over the years, you inevitably gain a sense of proportion, appreciating the depths of each experience and commitment.

FEED THE HABIT:

Identify your priorities. Too many people hit their later years and think, "I've fought all the wrong battles. Now look where I am." Identify your values, create your priorities, and make those the dynamic template for how you live your life and love the people close to you.

Keep a daily battle log. Divide your log into sections devoted to each of your daily relationships. These might include your partner, child, boss, best friend, etc. When you pick a battle by making a demand, setting a condition, or offering a criticism, write it down. Note what it was and how you presented it. Examine the results at the end of each day. Push yourself by limiting yourself to one (yes, one) battle a day. If you chose to make an issue of the toothpaste cap off the toothpaste, you've filled your quota for the day, and you're done no matter what other significant issues come up. Use the exercise to learn to lead with your priorities.

Cultivate a new dimension. How much of your happiness is controlled by other people? No one is happy all the time, but do you have a foundation that centers you and offers you emotional stability, no matter what your surrounding circumstances? If you keep yourself on secure emotional ground, you're better able to lead with your ultimate priorities and to be in richer, more genuine relationships with other people.

 # GET OVER IT

The hunter-gatherer society certainly saw its measure of conflict and revenge, but it was also the breeding ground for our capacity to forgive. Michael E. McCullough, author of *Beyond Revenge: The Evolution of the Forgiveness Instinct*, explains that the ability to forgive is as much a result of natural selection as the impulse for revenge. It's a practice that's been observed in nearly every human society and in other animals, including chimpanzees, which offer soothing sounds and touch following antagonistic confrontations. Forgiveness, McCullough suggests, likely evolved as a means of social cooperation: "By forgiving and repairing relationships, our ancestors were in a better position to glean the benefits of cooperation between group members—which, in turn, increased their evolutionary fitness."[6]

The fact is, a band member who wouldn't give up a grudge would've been a serious drag on the rest of the group. If he couldn't learn to let it go, he probably would've been out of the picture before too long. There just wasn't room for festering negative emotions that eroded the community. Band life was

YOU ARE HARDWIRED *to conserve energy and minimize personal risk.*

MODERN DISCONNECT: *abundance of choices.*

PRIMAL CONNECTION: *know when to say no and walk away.*

flexible, and individuals occasionally left (or were forced to leave) because of social conflict. However, being shunned or choosing to leave at an inopportune time in the season left a person extremely vulnerable. The risk just wasn't worth the emotional indulgence. Put simply, a thick skin would've been beneficial to survival.

> ❝ **The hunter-gatherer society certainly saw its measure of conflict and revenge, but it was also the breeding ground for our capacity to forgive.** ❞

Without this traditional imperative to *let it go*, we moderns too often indulge in wallowing—to our own detriment. How many people walk around living "half-lives" because so much of themselves is entangled in the bramble of past hurts, offenses, and travails? How many years will they allow themselves to be stuck there? What will they miss out on in the meantime?

Forgiveness isn't just about the other person's wellbeing. It's ultimately about your own. You're cutting the present loose from the past. You're putting yourself in charge of your own emotional health instead of letting someone else dictate it each day of your life. Research shows that people who forgive are more satisfied with life, and experience fewer feelings of emotional distress. Likewise, if you're the one who made a mistake and are still suffering the emotional toll, accept that it's time to move forward. Take responsibility, choose to live in integrity with yourself and others. Every day you let another person—or past mistake—control your wellbeing is a day you miss living fully.

In addition to releasing the significant resentments from your past, learn to let go of the smaller daily conflicts that build up with the people in your life—your significant other, children, co-workers, and friends. Imagine the individual peace and relationship potential that you might gain with a shift in your emotions.

FEED THE HABIT:

Learn to recognize negative self-chatter. When you start to go down the emotional road of replaying negative experiences, change the recording. We all do it at some point—mulling every nuance of a past failure, recalling every wrinkle of negative interactions. Cultivate the discipline to stop yourself mid-thought and diffuse the angry, fight-or-flight hormonal cascade before it overtakes you. Identify the physical feelings and mental associations that set it all in motion. Consciously stop the thought and step back from the precipice. Relax and redirect.

Use ritual to create emotional closure. There's an old New Year's tradition (attributed to a number of countries) of opening the front door at midnight to sweep out the old and let in the new. It's a meaningful metaphor in choosing forgiveness. Some people write down their thoughts about the past and burn them to make manifest the letting go of the old—disappointments, regrets, grief, and even joys. The idea here is to create the mental space that allows you to be fully present in the now, in each new moment—to not be burdened by past defeats or grudges or relying on previous successes. Resolve each day to open up that door—to accept the past for all its good and bad and then let it go, to meet the new day with determination, optimism, and no excuses.

 # SHARPEN YOUR SPEAR

Anthropologically, *Homo sapiens sapiens* (i.e., modern humans) ultimately prevailed over the *Homo sapiens neanderthalensis* in the theater of evolution. Why? Despite all the badmouthing, Neanderthals weren't the dim, slow creatures they're often accused of having been. Anthropological evidence suggests they used hunting implements, made clothing, built shelters, and buried their dead. If Neanderthals had so much in common with *Homo sapiens sapiens*, what made the fatal difference? What did *Homo sapiens sapiens* have that they didn't? The answer: better tools, better skills.[7]

The two groups hashed out their existence (and evolutionary competition) in a descending Ice Age. The group that adapted the best won out, and the rest is history. *Homo sapiens sapiens* are thought to have been better foragers. They're known to have had the pivotal advantage of projectile weapons for hunting. Many experts believe they benefited from developing a more complex language ability. Despite having survived for more than 150,000 years in the relatively harsh climate of Europe, the Neanderthals succumbed when conditions took a turn for the worse. *Homo sap sap*, however, had what it took to make it through.

> **"** *Homo sapiens sapiens* (i.e. modern humans) ultimately prevailed over the *Homo sapiens neanderthalensis* in the theater of evolution. Why? **"**

Fast-forward to today, and we in the twenty-first century face a similar challenge of trying to make a living in ever-changing conditions. We aren't working with the long scope of evolution in our personal pursuits, but the general lesson holds: to get what we want, we must fashion a better spear. This can mean pushing yourself to new dimensions in your career. It can mean creating a job situation that allows you to live your values and offers you more flexibility. It can mean cultivating a sense of vocation outside of your specific profession. Ultimately, sharpening your spear is about developing yourself in satisfying, diversified ways that will help you experience success, however you conceive of it.

For most of us, a career easily consumes most of our time. We want that investment to offer something substantial and enriching to our lives. So, at the very least, we can bring a positive, primal attitude to subsistence. Instead of thinking of work as something you *have* to do, think of it as something you *get* to do. And that means you get to have your basic needs met. You get to put dinner on the table for ourselves and our families. That would've been enough for our hunter-gatherer ancestors to celebrate. When we lose sight of the basic value of our effort, we forget to experience the joy.

Many times—understandably—we want more from that investment. We're looking for a means of self-actualization. We're looking for intellectual challenge, social engagement, creative potential. Too often people go after the profession they think they're supposed to want—because of the paycheck, prestige, or apparent security. Others feel locked into a career because of age. This job is all they've ever done, and it must be too late to take on new ventures. Nothing could be further from the truth.

In traditional societies, men and women often take on new roles with age. Decide to own the self-knowledge that comes with age, and have the courage to invent a new and better path for yourself. Whatever stage in the game you're at, if you can choose a career that aligns with your passion, your professional path will offer fulfillment as well as prosperity. Developing a successful career, like creating a more complex projectile, takes time and dedication. Investing in a passion is a lot more motivating—and rewarding.

Either way, develop yourself broadly. "Specialization," as sci-fi writer Robert A. Heinlein once said, "is for insects." You're more than a single role, a discrete skill, a particular job. Our ancestors, by necessity, were Jacks and Janes of many trades. In a small band, it was too risky to turn over essential functions to an individual who may leave at the end of a migratory season (or be killed by a predator). It's a privilege this day and age to decide what is and is not worth your time, but there's something to be said for being well-rounded. Genius, for example, doesn't stem from the tunnel vision of specialization but from the innovative visualization of creative, unexpected connections. On more modest terms, simply having a whole host of skills can expand not only your self-sufficiency, but your sense of personal identity, competence, and resiliency.

FEED THE HABIT:

Take a class or attend a conference. Maybe it's a new dimension of your current profession or a new path entirely. Learn more about the scope of the field and the variety of positions in it.

Volunteer or take a side job. If your current job isn't your personal passion, try something on the side that feeds your interest.

Fill your free time wisely. Choose activities and social connections that enrich and expand your life. Read. Travel. Develop yourself through a hobby.

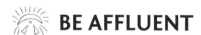 # BE AFFLUENT

Most of what we're taught about our hunter-gatherer forebearers suggests their lives were nothing but animalistic want and abject misery. Imagine, however, an existence raw yet less brutish than we've been taught, one that included periods of great abundance. This was the radical notion set forth by anthropologist

YOU ARE HARDWIRED *for vast amounts of downtime.*

MODERN DISCONNECT: *we get caught up in the busyness of life.*

PRIMAL CONNECTION: *reframe your definition of affluence.*

Marshall Sahlins in 1966, when he convincingly argued that our hunter-gatherer ancestors were the original affluent society.

Sahlin's anthropological analyses suggest we can estimate hunter-gatherers' daily foraging and food preparation time between two and six hours a day. Translation: vast amounts of leisure time!

So, how did they fill a typical day? Barring some apparent threat or dramatic weather incident, they'd likely take their time in the morning. What was there to rush to anyway? There might be talk of the previous day's activities or plans for an impending hunt. Some might draw water from a nearby stream. Children would play. Babies and toddlers would nurse. Those who were hungry right away

> **We can estimate hunter-gatherers' daily foraging and food preparation time between two and six hours a day. Translation: vast amounts of leisure time!**

could munch on remnants of the prior day's gatherings or lightly forage for a morning meal. A successful hunting day was enough to warrant an evening feast, followed later with bringing out drums, flutes, dried pods, and other instruments. They would sing. Many would dance. Other nights might bring well-known and welcome stories around the intimacy of a fire circle. Beyond the circle there would be little to watch on most nights but the stars and the dim silhouette of a darkening landscape, the nearby sound of the wind in the grasses and, in the distance, calls of animals.

Let me make it perfectly clear now that I'm not advocating that you quit your job, disavow your worldly possessions, join a commune, and walk around barefoot in a robe all day. (Well, the barefoot part would be OK.) I support working hard, competing in the free market, and contributing to the economy by producing and consuming goods and services to make for a better life for yourself and those around you. While there is opportunity for lively philosophical debate about the inequitable distribution of wealth, abuse of human and natural resources, and other flaws inherent with the modern global economy, I prefer that we focus here on broadening your perspective of wealth to include good health, creative freedom, job satisfaction, and deeply meaningful relationships with family and friends. Above all, I'd like to emphasize quality time.

THE ULTIMATE PRIMAL COMMODITY

At birth, we are bestowed with the gift of life, which, when you boil it all down, amounts to large a block of time. How we choose to spend this valuable gift is ours and ours alone. In our youth, we have little concept of time, perhaps as it should be, filling it with play, curiosity, and discovery. Yet as adults, when we're not logging in hours building a career, we fill it with undesired social obligations, full itineraries, and endless chores—tethered to status and possessions. Shouldn't our time be more enjoyable, more leisurely?

Sadly, too many ask themselves this question just as their time begins to markedly shrink, leaving them wondering if their days on this planet could have been better spent. It is only then they begin to appreciate the simplest of pleasures, those very things that had always been there but had typically been taken for granted.

When it comes to enriching experiences—quality time—what can our ancestors' example teach us? We sometimes imagine that if we could just "manage" our time and organize our lives better that we'll be happier and more relaxed. Maybe we need *less* to manage in the first place. (That goes double for the kids.) Do we truly need more impressive weekend plans? Maybe we should just spend more time sprawled out in the grass laughing with the kids or curling up with our partner. A Sunday afternoon nap is an underappreciated indulgence. How about lounging at the local beach or park—or enjoying a glass of wine sitting in the kiddie pool after the kids have gone to bed? These are simple but seemingly scarce luxuries these days. Try including more frequent pleasures in your life— ideally, fifty percent of your waking time. Yes, I know. That's a lot considering the typical forty-hour workweek. But there are ways, even during your rush-hour morning commutes, to grasp additional leisure time. Let's explore.

REFRAMING YOUR DEFINITION OF AFFLUENCE

Gratitude, with a capital G. The word should resonate as holy (which has the same root as healthy, and means whole), for without it, boredom prevails. With it, you *acknowledge* and *appreciate* life's gifts. This embodiment extends beyond your attitude to become an actual personality trait, a stress management tool, and an overall way of life. You live in gratitude because you are here today—appreciative of the lessons and journey of your past, however imperfect—for no other particular reason or caveat. And you remain in gratitude through the daily struggles that give meaning and richness to your life.

Our ancestors devised animism and deities to thank for the bounties in nature. More recently in our history, tribal societies such as the Native Americans and the !Kung Bushmen of southern Africa thank the animal's spirit for providing sustenance after it has been killed. If daily prayer or weekly services have a place in your life, you may be familiar with similar themes. But don't overlook other modest ways to show gratitude in your day-to-day life. Giving yourself the luxury of a warm bath, making a phone call to grandma, or presenting a home-cooked meal to your family all count, too, if your intention is in the right place.

When you practice an attitude of gratitude, you appreciate what you have, not envy what you lack. It means you're a good steward. You nourish and exercise your body and mind, cherish and respect your spouse, love your dog, keep your home clean and orderly, encourage your children. If you water your garden, you'll watch it grow.

It's the ability to see the beauty in simple things: a good red wine, a partner's intimate touch, that post-workout calm, a great night's sleep. The feel of the sun on your face, your feet in the wet sand, and your hands in the cool dirt. Or the thrill of pedaling down a rugged dirt trail, or the peace of floating on a quiet lake. Some time ago, for me, it was tasting the best shrimp of my life—grilled perfectly tender and flavorful in the shell with a mango-citrus dipping juice. Eating with my hands, sitting on the beach, enjoying the company of my wife and friends, I relished the full moment as much as that enticing platter.

When you practice gratitude, you create a happier take on your day-to-day world. But I am absolutely certain abundance only comes to people who appreciate the small gifts, the humble blessings, the basics. Oprah Winfrey is very much aware of this concept, saying it wasn't until she went to Africa and had to carry water for every use of it that she realized her good fortune. She has said she hasn't looked at water the same way again, never again has taken it for granted. Every time she turns on the tap, she is grateful.

Even material things, when combined with gratitude, multiply in value—your favorite T-shirt, your surfboard, your Ford Mustang. Practice gratitude regularly, make it a habit, and a curious thing begins to happen. Whether by an unscientific, mystical law of the universe, or simply by virtue of appreciating what you already have, you begin to open yourself to receive more. Such is the reward of good stewardship. And something else, even more curious: you actually find appreciation in some of life's bitterest pills. Maybe your upbringing was not that great. It gave you character, didn't it? So you got laid off? Great! You get an opportunity to explore a new adventure. Injured while training for your big marathon race? Ah, an opportunity to explore the novelty and fitness benefits of cross-training. Can you see how the more you appreciate, the more you see the glass half full rather than half empty, the more you *feel* gratitude—and you must feel it—the more aware you become of life's hidden gifts? Can you see how the more you appreciate, the *richer* you become?

But don't take my word for it. Let's look at the science: University of California, Davis professor Robert Emmons, editor-in-chief of the *Journal of Positive Psychology* and author of *Thanks!: How Practicing Gratitude Can Make You Happier*, believes that living in gratitude is the single quickest and most efficient pathway to becoming happier. Yes, Emmons and other leaders in the burgeoning field of positive psychology can actually quantify this stuff, asserting that while familial genetics plays a large role in longevity, researchers have amassed significant data suggesting that up to 75 percent of longevity is related to psychological and behavioral factors. Emmons notes that chronically angry, depressed, or pessimistic people have long been observed to have an increased disease risk and shorter life spans. However, those who kept a simple "gratitude journal" for three weeks or longer reported better sleep, increased energy, heightened creativity, enthusiasm, determination, and optimism ... and an increased desire for exercise. Now that's something to be grateful for!

KEEP IT SIMPLE

Gratitude gives way to simplicity, notes Sarah Ban Breathnach in *Simple Abundance*. Indeed, simplicity was the way of our ancestors, and they were richly rewarded for it. Owning *things* was not only irrelevant, but a hindrance to our ancestors' semi-nomadic life. They met their needs on a daily basis without concern for surplus or excessive material possessions, trusting that the natural environment would provide. Marshall Sahlins refers to this way of life as "affluence without abundance" (also the "Zen road to affluence"), for such a nonmaterialistic value system affords many luxuries, including devotion to family and clan.

If this sounds like an idealist's interpretation, consider the isolated hunter-gatherer societies across the globe today, who, like our ancient ancestors, work less, enjoy more leisure time, have no stress related to our Western mentality (i.e., the rat-race mentality) and enjoy arguably higher levels of life satisfaction in

> **" When you practice an attitude of gratitude, you appreciate what you have, not envy what you lack. "**

many enviable and profound ways. On a recent trip to South Africa, I witnessed this firsthand when we visited, by our materialistic standards, a dirt-poor village. The most memorable thing that came out of that experience for me was that everyone was smiling—*all the time.*

Not to discount the positive motivation of striving for career success and material gain (and the satisfaction that comes from succeeding), but we must also recognize the disadvantages of the modern mindset. Our culture, with its penchant for bigger, faster, stronger, tries to sell us the idea that the current more-is-better model is the norm, the inevitable, even the ideal. It's the path of progress, we're told, and we'd best keep up or get left behind. One can't help asking, the path to whose progress?

The advertising firms on Madison Avenue have created a new standard in our collective psyche, defining in the shallowest terms who we should be, how we should look, and what we should have. I'm reminded of the dialogue in a scene from the popular television series *Mad Men*, depicting the dog-eat-dog world of 1960s advertising:

Advertising is based on one thing: happiness. And you know what happiness is? Happiness is the smell of a new car. It's freedom from fear. It's a billboard on the side of the road that screams reassurance that whatever you are doing is OK. You are OK.

Again, I'm not asking you to disavow your worldly possessions. Only to take inventory of the superfluous "stuff": impulse buys and random things that strap you down with burden. If your world is cluttered with items that don't bring you security, happiness, beauty, or meaningfulness, you are most certainly weighed down. Not only do these things clutter your exterior world but your interior world as well. More to take care of, more to haul around, more to box up and keep in storage. Liberate yourself, and get rid of it. And from this point on, commit to quality over quantity. Or as the minimalists say, live with less but only the best. Yes, less really can be more.

FEED THE HABIT:

Celebrate life with affordable luxuries. Pull out your good china and silverware and light some long-stemmed candles … just because. Pick some flowers (or buy a cheap bouquet) and set them in your bedroom. Splurge on a basket of organic blueberries ($7 in some places!) or some fancy high-priced cappuccino. Use your imagination. What other ways can you find to indulge?

Start a gratitude journal. Make a comprehensive list of the things you are grateful for. See if you can list thirty, but strive for one hundred. I'll give you five right now: your senses of sight, hearing, smelling, feeling, and tasting. Run with it. And be sure to come back to your journal often to record new entries. I recommend daily.

Live within your means, lower if possible.

Make a personal visit, a phone call, or write a handwritten letter. Express your Gratitude to someone who deserves it, but hasn't been properly thanked.

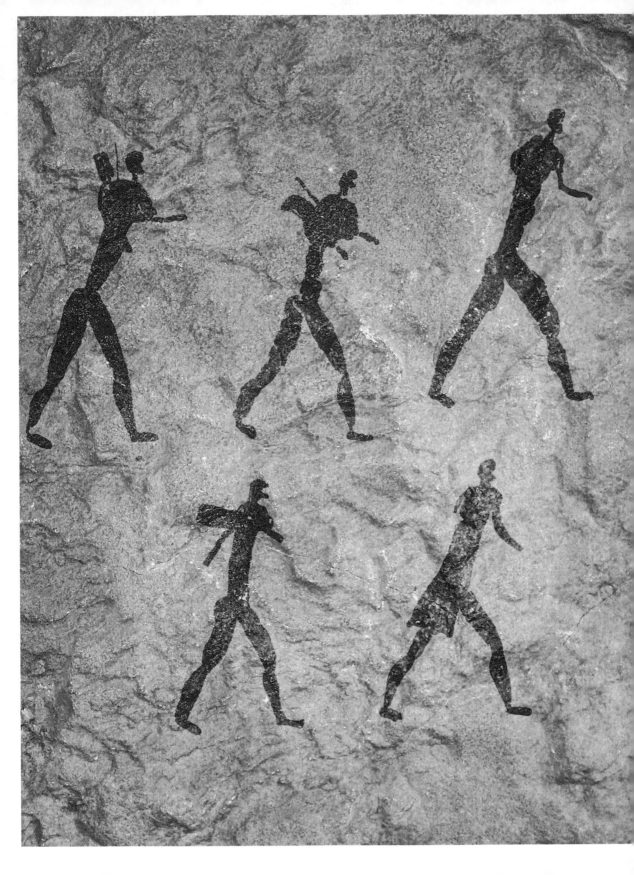

THE BODY CONNECTION

OUR BODIES EVOLVED TO BE seats of perception, intuition, and consciousness through which we sense, feel, think, and connect with the world. Indeed, the body is stunningly intertwined with the mind. The two influence one another in ways we're only now beginning to understand. Their communication is constant, nuanced, and bidirectional. While the basics of diet and exercise to achieve optimal gene expression were covered extensively in *The Primal Blueprint*, this section revisits the body connection to address the transformative power of human touch, how to transition to a barefoot-dominant lifestyle, and the importance of correct posture and biomechanics, and the dangers of a sedentary modern lifestyle. You will learn the correct way to sit, stand, and walk, and even why standing up at work can help you increase energy and burn body fat.

A touch is worth a thousand words any day.

ROBIN DUNBAR
ANTHROPOLOGIST

STAY IN TOUCH

THE LARGEST ORGAN OF OUR body is the skin. Its protective layers guard our muscles, bones, internal organs, and ligaments, while its active function results in the most fundamental of our five senses: touch. There is perhaps no more poignant, more visceral means of establishing connection than by way of this sense. It is the most primal, after all; the one developed first in the womb. We're hardwired to enjoy the neurochemical rewards for the positive touch we share with others—holding our children, embracing a friend, or caressing our partner. It's the primal way.

Social grooming, in fact, is utilitarian among many species. For one, not all animals can completely clean themselves alone. But more important, it reinforces social structure and interpersonal relationships. Wolf packs sleep nuzzled close together, and not just for warmth. Kangaroo kids hang out in that famous pouch. And apes will spend hours grooming each other. How about our pets? Dogs will nuzzle and lick their masters, and cats will head butt you and curl up in your lap and meow until you relent and offer your hand. It's almost like touch is a requirement of animals; they crave and need it. And so do we, though we may not always let on.

In traditional societies, however, touch plays a much more extensive role in interpersonal communication. This really hits home when I travel for business, and I'm away from my family and close friends. It's during these times that I realize just how ubiquitous our self-made, imaginary personal bubbles have become. We all walk around with them. As the world becomes more and more crowded, we're somehow able to maneuver through it without so much as touching a single person unless we're crammed into a train or city street. And still, even in those situations, people are loathe to make contact with one another—even ocular—and we manage to avoid most of it.

Take the phrase "touchy feely," for example. What imagery does it conjure? Its literal definition is "marked by or emphasizing physical closeness and emotional openness," but the phrase is commonly delivered as an epithet. Men disinclined to hug their fathers, their kids, or their male friends; young men and women unable to separate honest affection from sexual attention; children who spend their formative years touching the cold, hard plastic of an Xbox controller or remote control without developing nary a scrape, bruise, or welt from physical contact with peers; entire families that text, chat, or email to communicate, even when living under the same roof, this is the legacy of our apparently social disfavor—even revulsion in some cases—for physical closeness.

It starts with infants, of course. Many babies, upon being born, are instantly whisked away for checkups, tests, and to "let the mother rest." It seems odd that in that most crucial of windows, where the mother-child post-womb relationship is in its infancy, many kids don't even get to see their mothers. Instead, they're in some room with some stranger performing odd things on them.

As mentioned, the first sense infants develop in the womb is touch, and when they're born, touch is the most pre-attuned sense, whereas the senses of sight and taste take months to develop fully. A just-born infant needs to feel the warmth of his or her mother, and she in turn needs the baby's. Newborns need to indulge the only viable sense available at the moment. Being placed on mom's chest right after birth, the newborn's temperature regulates with her body heat. The baby's heart rate and oxygen intake stabilizes. The skin-to-skin contact triggers a powerful cascade of chemical

YOU ARE HARDWIRED *to give and receive human touch.*

MODERN DISCONNECT: *overly formal customs and self-made, imaginary personal bubbles.*

PRIMAL CONNECTION: *make hugs your default greeting, cuddle your family, pet animals, give and receive massage ... and don't forget sex.*

responses that includes foremost oxytocin, a neuropeptide associated with trust and bonding.

Oxytocin is a primary factor in our evolution as a social species. It brings us—and keeps us—together in long-term pair bonds. It motivates us to care for our offspring through lengthy (and trying) childhoods. An emotional as well as evolutionary force, oxytocin is a potent neurohormone that has the power to shift—or even build—our individual capacity for and disposition toward social interpretation. The more oxytocin we have running through us, the more connected, trusting, and cared for we generally feel.

> ❝ Skin-to-skin contact triggers a powerful cascade of chemical responses that includes foremost oxytocin, a neuropeptide associated with trust and bonding. ❞

Newborns who have abundant contact with their caregivers, particularly the mother, each day tend to be calmer and less fussy. They tend to sleep better and fall into a regulated schedule more easily than those who receive less touch. They gain weight and grow more. On the other hand, babies who experience touch deprivation show markedly suppressed levels of growth hormone, oxytocin and vasopressin (another bonding-related hormone), and higher levels of cortisol (the primary neurochemical associated with stress). Such was the case with the children found living in institutionalized Romanian orphanages a few decades ago following the fall of communism.[1] The impact of early touch deprivation distorted their hormonal profile years after they'd been adopted into caring homes.

Just as the mother of a newborn feels the surge of oxytocin that will encourage her to bond with her child and nurture him, we garner the same feel-good hormonal benefits when we hug a dear friend. A caring touch offers a boost of oxytocin that can lower our stress hormone levels as well as blood pressure.[2] Research shows it can even act as a buffer for the stressful experiences we face. One study suggests even thinking about touch from our partners, for example, is enough to raise oxytocin levels and calm us.[3]

Because touch helps regulate cortisol and can induce the body's relaxation response, it also results in a heightened immune function. Massage recipients in studies also show a reduction in the inflammatory cytokines that are often seen in autoimmune disorders.[4] Furthermore, they exhibit approximately a 30 percent increase in serotonin and dopamine levels (although basic touch appears to raise serotonin and dopamine levels as well).[5] Moreover, supportive and therapeutic massage can dampen the perception of pain associated with everything from childbirth to cancer to fibromyalgia.

In its immense and confounding subtlety, touch helps us read the cues of both our physical environments and our social relationships. Whether it's carrying your baby in a sling, enjoying skin-to-skin contact with your lover, high-fiving your teammates, or hugging a friend you encounter on the street, touch spans the scope of human social identity and interaction. It's a silent but potent language with the power to comfort, heal, provoke, or even persuade us. Touch is a well to be filled—each and every day. Look for chances to expand your experience of touch. Let your guard down and get creative. Here are a few ideas to get you started:

Hug the people you love (and see) the most. With our busy schedules, we can pass by our partners with barely anything but a quick kiss on the way out the door. Reclaim cuddling with your little ones. Pile in the bed close and cozy for storytime. Use a sling or co-sleep safely with babies. As much as he grimaces, hug your grumpy teenager. (He needs and wants his parents' loving touch despite his claims to the contrary.) And don't forget your partner. Trade the quick goodbye peck for a real hug, a passing touch on the shoulder for holding hands, or offer a back rub out of the blue.

Make hugs your default greeting. Some of us come from touchy-feely families and incorporate the same pattern into our friendships. We hug and kiss one another whether it's been nine months or nine hours since we saw each other last. Others among us need to learn the habit. Our inclination to touch one another, of course, is culturally influenced. (Lucky are the citizens of European cultures, who frequently greet both genders with a kiss to each cheek.) Consider it an investment in your relationships and wellbeing to offer hugs, hand holding, and other supportive touch to friends and extended family. Especially for older, less socially connected relatives, your touch may be the only contact they experience in a day—or a week. Honor their humanity as well as your own by giving them an extended and earnest embrace.

Pet animals. They don't call them pets for nothing. Your golden retriever or calico experiences a boost in bonding, and so will you when you take the chance to pet them and show you care. Countless studies demonstrate the calming affect of petting animals—a slower heart rate, lower blood pressure, moderated cortisol. Let's face it: there's no emotional baggage or ambiguity with animals as there can be with people. There's nothing but loyalty and appreciation when you offer your pet some loving strokes or a hug. If you don't have a pet of your own, offer to "animal-sit" for a neighbor's pet or volunteer at an animal shelter where they often need people to play with and walk animals.

Use subtle touch in passing interactions. Resolve to use subtle (and appropriate) touch with more casual acquaintances or even strangers in your day. Lightly touch a person's arm as you excuse yourself to the bus seat behind them or a coworker's elbow as you greet them while passing through the office. Notice how these subtle gestures bring about smiles and improve the dynamics of communication. But don't force it. Take advantage only of *natural* opportunities for touch, and pay attention to cues of receptiveness from others.

Don't forget about sex. Full skin-on-skin contact is the perfect scenario for boosting your oxytocin among other feel-great endorphins. Sex supports your bond with your partner neurochemically. Add to this the apparent immune benefits. In one study, subjects who had sex once or twice a week showed 30 percent more IgA.[6] Animal research even suggests sex increases cell proliferation in the brain's hippocampus.[7]

Get a massage. Research shows a professional massage boosts immune response. It truly is an art that's well worth the investment whenever you can swing it.[8]

*Forget not that the earth delights to feel your bare feet
and the winds long to play with your hair.*

KAHLIL GIBRAN

GO BAREFOOT!

IF OUR GENES EXPECT ANYTHING from us, it's that we ought to be barefoot most of the time. After all, the bipedalism that helps define our species—a trait we've spent seven million years perfecting—depends on our feet having a direct connection with the ground. Yet, when was the last time you walked barefoot? I'm not talking about a few yards from the shower to the bedroom. I mean when was the last time you went for a real stroll—on the beach, at the park, or even on smooth pavement—sans shoes? For most people over the age of ten, it's probably too long to even remember. Disconnect alert—and this time I mean it literally! We're disconnected from the earth and from the critical balance and biofeedback provided by our bare feet when we stand, walk, and especially run barefoot.

The fact is, shoes are viewed as a symbol of civilization, the obligatory accoutrement to our daily attire. However, the Primal camp views them as the quintessential example of how innovation can compromise physiological common sense. On top of all the gel inserts, padded cushions, arch supports, insoles, and orthotics, we bring endless cultural and social baggage to the adornment and protection of our feet. We try every heel height and incline, every footbed contour and toe box, every shaped style, material, and construction—all in the interest of outdoing (or thumbing our noses at) nature's original design.

Folks, we pay a major price in doing so—with lower back pain, skewed postural alignment, reduced hip mobility, and atrophied, imbalanced muscles. For a culture that hangs on every subsequent innovation, it would behoove us to realize that not every development springs from good science or rational enlightenment. Sometimes the simplest answer really is the best one.

> ## " We evolved to walk, hike, sprint, and even run long distances barefoot. "

At first blush, pursuing the barefoot connection may seem counterintuitive. The very idea of taking your feet out of their high-tech, protective cocoons to help relieve pain and lessen impact trauma ranks right up there with such radical (but accurate) advice as "Eat more fat to lose weight," and "Slow down your endurance workouts to get fit." But barefoot living has a proven track record. Barefoot enthusiasts, particularly those who previously responded poorly to conventional treatments, report relief from foot and lower extremity pain.

So, what exactly makes shoes such a problem? The human foot is a sensitive, capable, highly mobile appendage packed with an intricate network of bones, fascia, muscles, tendons, ligaments, and nerve endings, all of them charged with the awesome job of reacting to the environment they come in contact with, and constantly relaying that critical data to your brain to help you walk, stand, and run gracefully. Every footfall should inform your brain how to adjust to the shock and how to react to the change of terrain. This is the result of 2.5 million years of evolutionary design.

Slap your shoes back on and—presto!—nearly all of that sensory biofeedback vanishes. It's difficult to appreciate or respect the depth of this message, or even describe in words what a huge deal the shoe disconnect represents, especially when your perspective has been warped by a lifetime of having both of your feet essentially encased in casts. Have you ever broken your arm or wrist, been in a cast for six weeks, and then removed the cast to discover a withered appendage that seems completely out of sync with your nervous system and skeleton? Multiply the broken arm effect exponentially, and you can empathize with the long, painful prison sentence your feet have endured.

Skeptical? Try this: while standing in shoes, try to balance on one leg ... with your eyes closed! You lose your balance. Now try the same exercise barefoot. Notice how efficiently and dynamically your arch, individual toes, and heel bone absorb and disperse your center of gravity through subtle muscle contractions and weight shifts? This is how your feet, literally the foundation of your body, work to keep you in balance.

Next, go outside and run your toes and feet through the grass, sand, pebbles, what have you. Stand on bare pavement, even. Wiggle your toes and just feel. It's like awakening a thousand points of sensation. There's something so good, so luxurious about such a simple experience.

Can you imagine a more symbolic reconnect than allowing your body to engage with the earth on every step you take? We evolved to walk, hike, sprint, and even run long distances barefoot (or, more recently in our long history, sporting no more than rudimentary sandals, moccasins, or other similar protection). Going barefoot supports a feeling of emotional and spiritual grounding as well as literal grounding. In fact, one of the principles of Eastern philosophy states that your vital energy, a concept known as *chi*, will increase when your feet absorb energy directly from the earth. Chinese medicine places great emphasis on the bottom of the foot, where many organ energy meridians and acupressure points are located. Regardless of how philosophical you'd like to get about junking your clunkers for a barefoot walk in the park, you obtain a richer sensory experience when you negotiate varied surfaces, temperatures, and textures barefoot, and you automatically improve technique too.

Though our ancestors could probably walk twenty-five miles barefoot over rough ground without pain or problem, we must gradually integrate a barefoot experience to minimize injury risk. We face a more delicate process, since our dogs have likely atrophied greatly due to the long spell in solitary confinement. And a cold-turkey rejection of footwear, based on principle alone, might not fly for any other situation than a walk around the block right now. But that's OK. We'll proceed gradually and with caution.

Of course, we must also have to respect the constraints and conventions of the workplace and

YOU ARE HARDWIRED *to receive biofeedback from your bare feet.*

MODERN DISCONNECT: *restrictive, cushiony shoes with elevated heels and arch supports.*

PRIMAL CONNECTION: *tear off your shoes, toss aside your socks, and go barefoot.*

> ❝ **Going shoeless helps strengthen the muscles found in your feet, hips, and legs that aren't used when you wear shoes.** ❞

social customs (no shirt, no shoes, no service). And then we have sidewalks and parks sprinkled with bits of broken glass, motor oil stains, dog poop, and other hazards that pose a problem. But there is plenty of potential to enjoy the benefits of the barefoot connection—even for those residing in the most challenging environments. We'll soon be delving into the merits of *minimalist footwear*. But for now, let's consider the following points:

1. The elevated, softened heel support found in most shoes impedes our natural gait and can result in a shortened Achilles tendon and calf muscle.
2. Going shoeless helps strengthen the muscles found in your feet, hips, and legs that aren't used when you wear shoes. This in turn can increase coordination, agility, and balance.

And when you add exercise …

3. Running barefoot takes upwards of 4 percent less energy than running with shoes. You're relieved of that extra effort that goes into lugging the extra weight of even lightweight-style running shoes. Phew!
4. Running shoes encourage—perhaps even force you—into an inefficient heel-first landing with each stride. Can you imagine running heel to toe without shoes? You wouldn't do it. It would be much too traumatic. Landing on your heel results in undue shock and potential injury to your knees and back. It also results in an inefficient distribution of your center of gravity.
5. Running shoeless helps to improve your running technique. The natural and most effective way to run, as exemplified by top marathon runners, is to stride with a balanced center of gravity. Here's how: land on your midfoot with your bodyweight balanced and vertical from head to toe. Then push off quickly with light, smooth strides. This allows your arch, your Achilles tendon, and indeed the entire structure of your foot to act like the powerful natural catapult that it is.

6. Running barefoot prevents injury. When you run barefoot, you automatically achieve a light, efficient stride that balances center of gravity—*because it feels comfortable!* The cushy landing afforded by shoes lets you plod along with inefficient weight distribution and alteration of your center of gravity on each step. Multiply that by the 55,000 steps that you need to complete a marathon, and we're now talking about an overuse injury in the making!

GOING MINIMALIST

My barefoot journey began in 2006, when I stumbled upon rumblings on the Internet from grassroots enthusiasts proclaiming that a shoe revolution was "afoot." I've spent a fair amount of time working out and relaxing barefoot by virtue of living near the beach for the past few decades, so I was sold on the concept immediately. Going barefoot is so simple, so natural, and the positive feedback so immediate, that it was only a matter of time before the outdated bigger-is-better footwear philosophy of the fitness world would be seriously second-guessed.

Seven years later, it's gratifying to notice a strong mainstream barefoot movement happening today. In fact, the endurance-running community is aggressively rethinking its most elementary rule: all you need is a pair of stable, cushioned shoes. The desperation of suffering from recurring overuse injuries, despite doing the "right thing"—as dictated by conventional wisdom—has driven many to look outside the shoebox for answers. The answer being barefoot!

That said, I'm not a fan of tracking the likes of motor oil and other contaminants everywhere with me. Enter minimalist footwear.

The fast-growing minimalist footwear market gives you many options for fashion, function, and leisure, and you can certainly do well on a limited budget. Having several minimalist shoe options in your closet for various occasions—workouts, workplace, or trips to the supermarket—will help you conveniently grab precious barefoot time as you make your transition into a barefoot-dominant lifestyle. In the early years of my barefoot transition, I carried a pair of Vibram FiveFingers in my backpack on long hikes. When gentle sections of the trail came along, I switched my big shoes for the Vibrams for a half-hour or so. This strategy gave my body a chance to adapt to a barefoot experience with the security that I could return to big shoes before overstressing my still-sensitive feet. Of course, once I fully adapted, I threw the boots away forever. Let's take a look at some of the minimalist footwear options available:

Barefoot-simulation. Vibram FiveFingers shoes provide the most authentic barefoot experience available in footwear, thanks to a patented individual toe compartment design. They're offered in an assortment of models, ranging from the original, bare-bones classic to newer, beefed-up designs with carbon fiber–reinforced soles that allow for more rugged and versatile use. Not exactly cheap, FiveFingers retail between $80 and $120 per pair. But they are absolutely the way to go for workouts, hikes, and other outdoor activities. Beware of counterfeits, which are becoming a serious problem.

Dress shoes. When you must follow the crowd and wear dress shoes, choose the least heel-to-toe elevation possible. Feelmax, Terra Plana, and Tod's are some of the many interesting brands you might discover with minimalist styles. Visit BarefootMotion.com for a variety of minimalist footwear options for work, formal, and leisure wear.

Leisure. Try to go barefoot around the house when weather permits, or use reinforced socks (check out Injinji.com for their patented toe socks—they even work inside Vibrams!) or house slippers with minimal construction for cold weather. For warm weather, a basic pair of flip-flops or the more fancy Luna Sandals are great options for running errands or general leisure-time use. The key here is minimal heel-to-toe elevation.

Outdoor activity. Neoprene water socks, available at most sporting goods stores, offers inexpensive protection against the elements, with minimal construction and near-zero elevation of heel over midfoot.

Running. Minimalist shoes have gone mainstream! Depending on your transition level, the newer models from familiar brands could serve as good intermediate shoes as you move from restrictive to minimalist on the barefoot spectrum. The New Balance Minimus is a popular model, offering a "closer-to-barefoot" experience with a minimal heel elevation, flexible lightweight construction, and soles made by Vibram. Merrell Barefoot features a traditional single toe box and form-fitting Vibram soles. Lightweight racing flats provide minimal heel rise and a flexible sole. The Nike Free models have flexible soles and minimal heel counter support, but most come with the traditional elevated heel. Other brands to consider include ECCO's Biom line, Luna Sandals, Newton Running, and RunAmocs.

HOW TO GO (BACK TO) BAREFOOT

Grok went barefoot (or virtually barefoot) all day for his entire life, and consequently sported magnificently strong and durable feet capable of weathering myriad climates, terrains, and physical challenges. Going barefoot demands increased range of motion, muscular strength, and flexibility. In your quest to honor the design of your feet, certain strengthening and stretching exercises are necessary. These will help minimize any injury risk that might come as you transition to a barefoot lifestyle, in particular, the elimination of artificial support for your arches that cause the Achilles tendon to elongate.

Even though the Achilles tendon is the thickest and strongest tendon in the body, it is, due to underuse and atrophy, fragile. Similarly, our extensive reliance on arch-supporting shoes has made plantar fasciitis, a painful inflammation of the arch and heel area, one of the most common foot maladies. Plantar fasciitis—a painful, burning irritation of the heel—happens to those who wear bulky, elevated shoes as well as to those with ill-prepared feet attempting to integrate more barefoot time. The traditional prescription for plantar fasciitis—rest and *more* arch support via supportive shoes or custom-made orthotics—has not proven to be very successful. For many with overuse injuries, rest can cause further atrophy of the relevant tendons and muscles, and does nothing to address the underlying cause of the injury. Trust me, I have been there and done that!

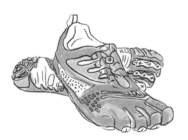

The barefoot connection is about addressing the *cause* of chronic pain and injuries by re-enabling the

Minimalist footwear, such as Vibram FiveFingers, protects bare feet while simulating a barefoot experience.

THE MIGHTY ACHILLES

The Achilles tendon may have been a weak spot for the Greek soldier, but scientists believe that it's the key to human running prowess and one of the major distinguishing characteristics of humans branching out from other African apes. Chimpanzees, gorillas, and other primates in our extended family tree lack a robust Achilles tendon or a prominent arch. Consequently, they are at a disadvantage for both sprinting and long-distance running.

Noted British computational primatologist Bill Sellers believes that the development of our strong Achilles tendons was our primary evolutionary adaptation![9] He suggests that they increased top human running speed by over 80 percent due to their ability to store "elastic energy" (our arches do this also), and therefore allowed humans to become hunters instead of herbivores. The resulting nutrient-dense diet afforded us with a more complex brain development. Still intent on running in those clunky, elevated-heel, motion-control shoes?

feet and lower extremities to function as nature intended—outside the confines of restrictive footwear. As we've discussed, this process is not guaranteed smooth sailing. There is a learning curve. In fact, somewhat of a tug-of-war will occur during your barefoot efforts. When you place muscles and tendons under exercise stress, they heat up, loosen up, and pump up with blood in response to the challenge. However, if your initial foray into the barefoot lifestyle is too ambitious, you will experience inflammation, tightening, and stiffness in the aftermath. In a condition such as plantar fasciitis, the tightened muscles pull at insertion points, causing pain in affected tendons and joints.

While I'm not a big proponent of aggressive stretching programs, certain targeted stretches can help you pull that tug-of-war rope back into balance, and help lengthen affected muscles and tendons so they become more resilient to barefoot living. Bear in mind, too, every time you walk around barefoot you are already getting a highly effective stretch and strengthening effect. As a result, consider stretching supplemental to your primary objective of gradually increasing the amount of time you spend barefoot or in minimalist footwear.

These exercises can be conducted anytime, following a brief warm-up of gentle movement to get the blood flowing in your lower extremities. The list is intended as a simplified, all-purpose program to lengthen the muscles and joints affected by a barefoot transition. In a short time, you will notice increased general flexibility and strengthened lower extremities. If you have specific injuries or medical conditions, please seek professional support to obtain a customized strengthening and stretching program.

Think about your walking form. It's important to have a few ideas about barefoot walking before actually kicking off the shoes and heading out. My basic foundation for barefoot walking? Take shorter strides and land softly; avoid overstriding and harsh, jarring footfalls.

Invest in a lacrosse ball. The plantar fascia, located on our feet, supports the arch and can get notoriously tight and unresponsive after a lifetime of shoe wearing. Likewise, our calves are likely unaccustomed to absorbing the impact of a footfall. Something as simple as a lacrosse ball can help reduce tightness in these areas and ease the transition.

For the fascia, place a lacrosse ball (a golf ball works fine, too) on the floor, rest one foot on top of it, and roll the ball around. Just explore your foot with the ball. It'll be painful at first, but that's how you know it's working. Roll each foot twice a day for about five minutes. Be sure to flex your foot and move your toes around as you roll over tight spots—try to put your foot through every possible range of motion it might see in the real world. To roll the calf muscles, sit on the ground with your leg outstretched, place the ball beneath your calf, and move the ball back and forth along the length of your lower leg. When you hit a tight spot, flex and extend your ankle until it starts to feel less tight. Be sure to hit every aspect of your calf. Roll each calf once a day for about five minutes.

Start slowly. When you start walking barefoot, keep it short. Slow linear progression is your friend here, especially if you've spent decades with your feet encased inside shoes—you no doubt have a great deal of atrophied muscles and tendons to rebuild. Don't risk failure by rushing the process. Do a ten-minute walk, max, on flat ground such as the sidewalk or a running track. You're sending some very strong, extremely new messages to your nervous system, feet, and legs, and you don't want to overwhelm the physical structures before they're ready. Give your connective tissue the chance to adapt and recover. The next time you walk, add ten more minutes. Maintain this progression until you're up to an hour and it's easy and effortless. When adding more time doesn't result in sore feet, calves, or legs, you're ready for new terrain. If you're headed out for an extended walk, however, take a pair of trusty shoes along with you … just in case.

Sample new ground cautiously. The beauty of walking, hiking, and running barefoot is that you get to experience the ground in an entirely new way. When you're wearing shoes, everything feels the same. You might notice big topographical changes, but you miss the little things. You miss the blades of grass between your toes, the way gravel sort of massages your soles, the way scalding sand gives way to cool, damp sand at the beach. Going barefoot, you have a new sensory front to consider. Eventually, this will give you greater mobility, stability, and control over your body, but it can also throw you off and lead to missteps (or even injuries) when you're just starting.

Be aware of the ground on which you walk. Look for rocks, sticks, and other sharp things. In time, you will glide across the ground effortlessly, subconsciously integrating the sensory input from your feet, but not yet. For now, you have to focus on your underfoot surroundings. Over time, that focus will come to you naturally—the way it was always intended to be.

DID YOU KNOW?

That each foot consists of twenty-six bones? Combined, your feet make up nearly a quarter of the total number of bones in your entire body. (The human skeleton contains 206.) When functioning optimally, your feet provide excellent balance, stability, impact absorption, weight transfer, and propulsion by aligning your knees, pelvis, spine, and upper body.

This awareness itself comprises its own metaphor, really. Consider it a chance to get out of your head and take a break from the endless cacophony of mental chatter. Quiet your mind. Put your focus in the here and now. Absorb the sensory experience. Be in your environment, and attend to your body's motion within it.

STRENGTHEN YOUR FEET

As you move into frequent barefooting, your feet will naturally grow stronger. Daily foot exercises will help move along the process. With a little practice and some strategic moves, you'll be as good as our ancestors in no time.

Toe spreads. Loop a rubber band around your toes, tight enough so that it pushes your toes together if you let it. Now, spread your toes out and hold that position for a few seconds. Do two sets of ten reps with each foot.

Toe squeezes. Stick pencils, fingers, or anything that can fit in between each toe and squeeze them together. Hold the squeeze for a few seconds before releasing. Do two sets of ten squeezes with each foot.

Toe points. Pick something in the room and point at it with your toe. Hold the position for five seconds, then reverse the direction and point your toes toward your face. Hold the position for five seconds. Repeat the process ten times with each foot.

Side roll. Stand up and slightly bend your knees. Roll onto the outer edges of your feet, take a few steps forward, then a few steps back to your starting spot. Roll back. Repeat for fifteen reps.

Sand walk. This obviously isn't available to everyone, but if you have access to sand, go for it. As you walk barefoot, squeeze the sand with your feet. Sand grabbing is an old trick for grip building, and the same concept applies to your feet. Consider it a good excuse to spend more time at the beach or a chance to make use of the kids' abandoned sandbox.

A good stance and posture reflect a proper state of mind.

MORIHEI UESHIBA

THE POWER OF POSTURE

JUST AS OUR GENES EXPECT us to walk upright and to go barefoot, they are also preprogrammed to expect a lifetime of pain-free movement through an almost infinite number of planes under various workloads. We are wired for the effortless attainment of perfect posture, yet poor posture and inefficient biomechanics are now commonplace in the industrialized world. We can blame a sedentary lifestyle, our excessive reliance on modern comforts (such as poorly designed chairs, braces that compensate for functional errors, and elevated shoes that compromise posture), and flawed cultural influences (such as slouching fashion models) for the pain and spinal degeneration that millions suffer from today. But it doesn't have to be this way. You can easily correct poor posture with a few simple lessons that can pave your way to a lifetime of pain-free activity.

The very obvious downside to poor posture is the chronic and often debilitating physical pain that accompanies it. If you spend your days sitting, standing, and walking with a fundamentally flawed posture, it will catch up with you in the form of pain, increased injury risk, and long-term degeneration. If you want to live a long, active life, a healthy functioning spine is essential. The spinal cord is essentially a high-bandwidth system for the transfer of information between nerves, organs, and other parts of our anatomy. Misalignments of the

> **"One of the most common forms of bad posture is when the head juts forward instead of extending straight up from the shoulders."**

spine (aka subluxation) can constrict nerve pathways, leading to all sorts of muscle, joint, and circulatory problems.

One of the most common forms of bad posture is when the head juts forward instead of extending straight up from the shoulders. According to Rene Cailliet, professor emeritus of University of Southern California's physical medicine and rehabilitation program, this posture "can add up to 30 pounds of abnormal leverage, pulling the entire spine out of alignment and may result in the loss of 30 percent of vital lung capacity."[10] Think about what that means: a diminished lung capacity will reduce available oxygen to all other parts of the body, including major organs like the brain and heart. Nerves are compressed at multiple sites, and soon you're experiencing both pain within the head and at the base of the neck. You're also setting yourself up for later thoracic spine damage, a rounding of the upper spine also known as a "dowager's hump."

THE GOKHALE METHOD

As the Mark's Daily Apple community has grown in recent years, I've had the good fortune to associate with some of the world's leading health experts. These are forward-thinking individuals who are pursuing sensible health solutions and exploring beyond the confines and critical-thinking errors of conventional wisdom. One such pioneer is Esther Gokhale, a licensed acupuncturist who specializes in non-invasive cures and prevention for spinal pain and injury.

Gokhale's quest for a better way to approach posture started over twenty years ago. Her motivation was personal, having suffered from debilitating sciatic pain associated with a pregnancy, followed by an unsuccessful surgery for a herniated disc. Today, she runs the highly acclaimed Gokhale Method Institute in Palo Alto, California, which has been heavily praised by the

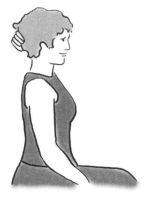

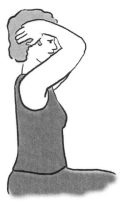

Straighten your neck

Option A: Grab a clump of hair at the base of your skull and gently pull it back and up.

Option B: Grasp the base of your skull with both hands and gently pull toward the top of your head.

Mayo Clinic, Stanford Medical Center, and the American Association of Orthopaedic Surgeons.

Gokhale's book, *8 Steps to a Pain-Free Back*, is filled with images of people from various regions of the developing world. These subjects exhibit efficient posture and biomechanics at rest as well as during arduous physical labor. One in particular shows a mother in the west African nation of Burkina Faso, walking barefoot with impeccable posture ... while balancing a large laundry load on her head with one hand, carrying a heavy bucket of supplies with the other hand, and, along for the ride, a baby nestled in a sling along her lower back. Talk about a lasting impression! No braces, no ibuprofen, no couch to collapse in at the end of the day—no problem, no complaints!

Meanwhile, here at home, we overindulge in modern comforts and sedentary lifestyles, and, as a result, suffer from chronic pain, muscle contraction (tightness), and inflammation. Your body initiates these symptoms, known as *adaptive protective mechanisms*, in an attempt to cope with the constant stress of poor posture and technique. Pain and muscle contraction inhibit your mobility while your immune system sends plasma proteins and leukocytes to the pain site to help accelerate the healing process. The excess fluid at the site of the injury is what produces the inflammatory swelling.

Popping a few pills when these mechanisms kick in overrides the body's desired effect—to get you to stop the damaging activity—and thus sets in motion a potentially endless cycle of further damage to your discs, nerves, tissues, and muscles. No wonder we see literally millions of folks dealing with chronic back and neck pain, and hundreds of thousands more undergoing major back surgery each year.

The ideal lower back *exhibits a mild groove with embedded vertebrae that appear as bumps and soft ridges on either side of the groove. A rounded lower back shows no groove and a swayed lower back displays a deep, exaggerated groove.*

The key to avoiding back pain (and achieving a healthy posture) boils down to *preserving a straight and elongated spine at all times.* This is true in all activities—standing, sitting, walking, sleeping, as well as physical work and complex athletics. Look at photos of weightlifters about to hoist the bar, basketball players in their defensive stance, baseball players awaiting a batted ball, football players in their three-point stance, or sprinters racing for the tape—in all cases they exhibit a straight and elongated spine as a component of correct technique. Millions, actually billions, of folks—physical laborers, current-day hunter-gatherers, repetitive task workers, and stooped-over field hands—in developing countries also exhibit characteristically excellent posture, and avoid injury while bending, lifting, pushing, and pulling.

According to Gokhale, the ideal is represented by a spine that is actually J-shaped if viewed from the side, not the more familiar S-shape we see in medical textbooks, conventional wisdom's representation of the ideal. Rather than ideal, it's simply the prevailing shape that has taken hold in modern society. Interestingly enough, Gokhale reports that in early twentieth-century medical textbooks, spinal models were more J-shaped, before the destructive effects of industrialized living and the 1920s' slouchy flapper fashion became the norm. In a J-shaped spine, the twenty-four bones (vertebrae) of the back are stacked in a straight line from the neck down through the lower back. The bottom of the spine curves slightly inward, forming a J shape from a side view. This is associated with a pelvis that is tipped slightly forward, or anteverted,

YOU ARE HARDWIRED *to sit, stand, and move with a straightened and elongated spine.*

MODERN DISCONNECT: *sitting, slouching, stooping, and slumping.*

PRIMAL CONNECTION: *relearn natural posture and biomechanics.*

which is ideal. Gokhale says an easy way to picture this is to imagine a beltline that is angled down towards the front. The result will position the buttocks behind the spine. Ready to try it out? First, slip off your shoes and anchor of your bodyweight on your heels. (Now you know why the calcaneous is such a dense bone!) Stand with feet comfortably shoulder-width apart, pointing forward or only slightly outward. Scrunch your toes inward to engage your arches. Beware the collapsed arch and outward-splaying feet that is both a cause and symptom of poor skeletal alignment. By engaging your arches and rocking your bodyweight back onto your heels, you should feel as though you have a strong, balanced base. Next, roll your shoulder blades, one at a time, into alignment on the same plane as your spine. To ensure your shoulders are positioned properly, turn your palms outward as you stand. This is a handy trigger to keep you honest and reprogram the common tendency to let the shoulders to cave forward and pull the head along too.

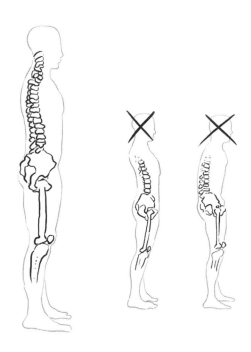

Standing with weight anchored on heels and shoulders aligned with spine, slightly contract only the upper level of your abdominal wall (i.e., the top level of your "six-pack"). This will keep you from collapsing your weight onto your spine and tucking your pelvis. Finally, reach up and grab a clump of hair at the back of your head and gently pull it back and up. This will allow your neck to elongate instead of the common compression that is associated with a protruding head. With neck elongated, your eyesight will project at a slight downward angle.

The J-shaped spine *of an antiverted pelvis (tipped slightly down) helps achieve a healthy posture. Conversely, a retroverted pelvis (tilted forward or tucked under) leads to tense muscles and slouching.*

As you engage with your new, correct posture, your entire body should feel relaxed and balanced. Refrain from the common corrective reaction of jamming the shoulder blades back unnaturally, which usually lasts only for the duration of the family holiday photo. While this overview of the basics can be valuable to overcome the most common error of protruding head, compressed neck, slouched shoulders, and a tucked-in pelvis, do yourself a favor and explore the Gokhale Method and *8 Steps to a Pain-Free Back* in greater depth—especially if back or neck pain is of particular concern to you.

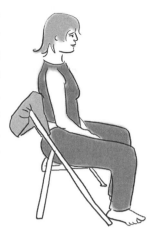

Stretchsitting
Push buttocks to back of chair with your feet hip-width apart. Lengthen your spine, eliminating any sway. Leave buttocks anchored to the chair, and relax the muscles of your torso, allowing the rib cage to separate as much as possible from the pelvis.

DON'T KNOW SQUAT

For millions of years, our ancestors never actually "went to the bathroom," because, well, the bathroom was pretty much right where they were. Turns out, our biomechanics evolved for us to defecate in a full squatting position, yet we insist on thwarting that most natural of urges by sitting on a porcelain device that interferes with proper elimination.

Unless you've traveled to a variety of Asian countries, you may never have seen nor tried a squatting toilet. (Picture a bowl below ground level for you to straddle—nothing more to it!) Many health and ergonomic experts—particularly in the Evolutionary Health movement—are passionately advocating the benefits of defecating in the squatting position and calling attention to an increasing amount of studies that confirm the health risks of using a sit-down toilet.

The commode came of age in the sixteenth century in the interest of giving royalty a little dignity while they did their private business. Then in the Victorian Age, the heyday of repressed social customs, came the invention of the flush toilet. As ordinary folks were able to utilize the invention across the industrialized British Empire, the "Emperor's new throne" became

YOU ARE HARDWIRED *to evacuate your bowels from a squatting position.*

MODERN DISCONNECT: *modern sit-down toilets that strain the bowels.*

PRIMAL CONNECTION: *use a step stool or other squat-aiding apparatus.*

yet another symbol of the mother country's smug superiority over their primitive colonials. Problem is, our bodies were designed for squatting not sitting.

When you defecate from a seated position, you pinch the angle between the rectum and the anus, leading to three times more straining and twice as long a time period to get the job done.[11] The inefficiencies and strain of sitting have been shown to increase the risk of constipation, hemorrhoids, hernias, diverticulosis (caused by excessive straining, believed to afflict half of all Americans aged sixty to eighty), uterine prolapse (which affects women during pregnancy and childbirth), and both urinary and anal incontinence.[12]

Surely all this talk of straining and pinching is unpleasant, but not as unpleasant as the serious health risks of using the everyday toilet. Because sitting inhibits a complete evacuation of the colon, residue can harden in a process known as fecal stagnation. Fecal stagnation causes colonies of harmful bacteria to take root in the contaminated areas, which has been linked to inflammation of the surrounding tissues and increased risk for colon cancer and inflammatory bowel diseases such as appendicitis, diverticulitis, ileitis, ulcerative colitis, irritable bowel syndrome, and Crohn's Disease. What's more, many of these bowel diseases are virtually unknown in developing countries, where squatting is used in lieu of the loo.

Squatting opens up the recto-anal angle (one study showed squatting affords an average angle of 132 degrees, and up to a completely straight 180 degrees, while toilet sitting results in an average angle of 92 degrees), offering your waste a path of least resistance for full evacuation.[13] Defecating in this position also strengthens the muscle fibers in your pelvic floor and protects the prostate, bladder, and uterine nerves from damage related to straining.

If you are interested in reduced constipation, less straining, and lower risk of inflammatory bowel conditions, squatting to eliminate is a connection with an obvious evolutionary precedent. And you don't need to move to Asia. There are a number of toilet stools available that will modify the position you adopt on a traditional toilet to enable the benefits of squatting. Visit SquattyPotty.com for a full education on the subject and direct ordering (units start at $35—cheaper than hemorrhoid surgery or colon cancer treatments).

Toilet squatting stools are U-shaped, so they slide around either side of your toilet bowl for easy storage. Slide the stool out a bit and you can rest your feet on elevated platforms, bend your knees, lower your torso between your thighs, and achieve a modified squatting position. After getting over your initial culturally influenced hesitations, you will realize how effortless and natural it feels to assume the squatting position, particularly when you use a specially designed stool.

Even if you are on the right track,
you'll get run over if you just sit there.

WILL ROGERS

MADE TO MOVE

FROM AN EVOLUTIONARY POINT OF view, exercise is even more essential than we've been told, but it doesn't have to be the mindless, miserable slogging people often think it is. Seen through the lens of our ancestors' lives, movement becomes layered with function, creativity, thrill, and play. Rather than some ancillary responsibility we pencil into our day, it's an indispensable dimension of a fully animated life.

The fact is we're meant to move and move often. Move in mundane ambulation as we go about the day's tasks. Move erratically and explosively as we push the boundaries of our limitations—because a life-threatening situation requires it, or because we crave the thrill to be found at the brink. Move creatively as we seek to express and experiment.

Movement feeds deeply ingrained instinct. What we often mistake for ennui in the modern age is, in part, a physical restlessness—like the detached, lost acquiescence of a caged animal. Movement, after all, defines us as humans. We're bipedal creatures who have evolved through both grand physical striving (e.g., migrating across the planet) and highly sophisticated endeavors (e.g., creating tools and technology). We relate to the world by acting upon it in some literal or figurative regard. Movement lives as motion and metaphor.

I've noticed something in the way people think about exercise. Sure, for some people it's simply about finishing the obligatory forty minutes on an elliptical. For others who readily embrace physical exertion, however, it's all about a different kind of goal—ambition and achievement. It's about the progression to a lower

> ## " What we often mistake for ennui in the modern age is, in part, a physical restlessness—like the detached, lost acquiescence of a caged animal. "

(or higher) weight, a faster time, or a longer run. I think that's part of being human—the drive to improve oneself. It's not everything, however. Humans are also adventurers and explorers. We're drawn by curiosity. We're moved by creative, seemingly arbitrary bouts of inspiration. The journey compels us, sometimes for no other reason than the journey itself with all its sights, sounds, and random incidents along the way. I think this applies to all aspects of living in the body—to movement, to sensing, and to play. We can embrace it also as a means of fulfillment and pleasure—with the power to reward us neurochemically and transform us epigenetically.

Beyond the full gamut of physical benefits, activity literally helps build and rebuild our brains as well as our muscles. Yes, exercise goes to the head in dramatically healthy ways throughout the course of a lifetime. There's truly no overselling this point. Most obviously, exercise increases blood flow to the brain, which provides more oxygen and energy but also reduces free-radical damage and enhances memory. Researchers also know that exercise stimulates the creation of new neurons and the production of brain-derived neurotrophic factor (BDNF), a chemical that's instrumental in neuron formation and preservation.[14] Then there's the impact on gene expression: exercise specifically

YOU ARE HARDWIRED
to move frequently at a comfortable pace.

MODERN DISCONNECT:
A sedentary lifestyle filled with prolonged sitting or standing.

PRIMAL CONNECTION:
move frequently and stand up at your desk!

> ## " While a devoted exercise regimen offers assorted benefits, it's simply not enough to protect you from the hazards of marathon sitting. "

promotes gene expression that supports plasticity,[15] the brain's crucial power to alter neural pathways, which allows us to adapt neurologically to and learn from our experiences. Plasticity is the stuff that fuels our cognitive development. There's no better way to maintain your intellectual faculties and adaptability than exercise.

DON'T BE AN ACTIVE COUCH POTATO!

Sitting is unnatural and uncomfortable for a species that has been standing, walking, and squatting for 2.5 million years. The human default resting position is actually squatting; it's only been in our very recent history that we've taken to marathon sitting. No wonder we contort and distort our bodies in vain attempts to avoid discomfort and pain while stuck in a chair!

So, what's so bad about sitting? For one, it weakens your gluteal muscles by deactivating them and putting them into a static stretch. Sitting also causes your hip flexors and hamstrings to shorten and tighten, gradually worsening over time. Unfortunately, strong glutes and good hip and hamstring mobility are critical to just about all manner of activity, from mundane daily tasks like picking up that paperclip off the floor to playing a demanding contact sport. If you are glued to the chair all day except for that lunchtime pickup basketball game or trail run, you can pretty much expect to get injured when you call upon your atrophied, imbalanced body for peak performance.

But far more sobering is the fact that scientists are now linking a sedentary lifestyle (defined as sitting for twenty-three hours a week or more) with diabetes, high blood pressure, cancer, cardiac disease, and premature death.[16] The physiology of inactivity theory suggests that prolonged sitting also causes weight gain by creating imbalances in critical metabolic hormones such as leptin, which regulates appetite and fat metabolism in the body. When leptin signaling is compromised, your brain will crave more food, and your body will default into a fat-storage hormonal pattern instead of a fat-burning hormonal pattern.[17] All this has scientists and members of the medical community repeating the same tagline: sitting is the new smoking.

There's even a new medical term associated with chronic sitting: active couch potato syndrome, used to describe people who suffer from the same health

EXERCISE AND THE AGING BRAIN

When it comes to the "aging brain," exercise rewrites the script on that notion. Not only is physical activity able to preserve brain function but it can also turn back the clock. As mentioned, exercise keeps the brain's stem cells working efficiently over the course of a lifetime and preserves brain tissue density.[19] The difference shows. When researchers scanned the brains of fifty-five subjects (ages fifty-five to seventy-nine), those with the most physically fit profiles (as measured by their maximal oxygen uptake) showed significant benefits in the frontal, temporal, and parietal regions of the brain, areas related to learning and memory functions.

The connection? Exercise stimulates the brain's release of "feel good" chemicals like endorphins that induce calm and contentment. (We could all use more of that.) It also supports the brain's efficient use of dopamine by increasing the number of receptors and the time dopamine remains in the synapses. Likewise, exercise has been shown to increase levels of the neurotransmitter gamma-aminobutyric acid (GABA) by influencing the brain's GABAergic system itself, which can reduce our "stress sensitivity and emotionality."[20] Low GABA levels are common in those with anxiety and mood disorders. Although exercise in general makes a positive impact, yoga in particular may hold special sway over GABA activity. According to a study published in *The Journal of Alternative and Complementary Medicine*, "asana" or pose-focused sessions resulted in more substantial improvements for mood and anxiety (and GABA levels) than a walking regimen did. I'd say it isn't only a reason to take up yoga but a reminder that our bodies benefit from a variety of movement experiences.[21]

risks as the absolute inactive despite devoting themselves to vigorous daily workouts—simply by virtue of the fact that they spend so much uninterrupted time sitting in long commutes, at desk jobs, and again when they get home and plop in front of the television. While a devoted exercise regimen offers assorted benefits, it's simply not enough to protect you from the hazards of marathon sitting.

By taking frequent breaks from sitting, however, even brief ones consisting of a minute or so, can measurably improve your circumstances. The moment you get up and get moving down the hall or around the office courtyard, you kick into gear the hormones—leptin, lipase, and insulin—that will shift you into a fat-burning mode. As endocrinologist James Levine of the Mayo Clinic explains:

> Simply by standing, you burn three times as many calories as you do sitting. Muscle contractions, including the ones required for standing, seem to trigger important processes related to the breakdown of fats and sugars. When you sit down, muscle contractions cease and these processes stall.[18]

One popular trend in Evolutionary Health circles is standup desks. You can create your own by retrofitting your computer desk with a couple of sturdy cardboard boxes. Nearly every member on staff at Primal Blueprint Publishing in Malibu independently transitioned to a predominantly standup workstation using this method. (Well, maybe a little peer and environmental influence was involved, but hey—that's a good thing!)

Standing at your work desk re-engages your muscles, promotes good posture, burns more calories, and generally avoids the perils of long periods in the chair. Standing also creates such metabolic efficiencies as increased calorie burning, improved circulation (including to your brain), and increased muscle recruitment. At first it may feel unnatural and uncomfortable to lose the chair, and you can certainly proceed with this exercise gradually. Stand for as long as you're comfortable, return to your chair for a sufficient rest period, then cycle into another standup period.

Even if you proceed with stand-and-sit cycles gradually, standing should predominate over sitting with a few months of effort. Let the transition happen at your own pace, and make sure you don't experience pain in your back or lower extremities from standing too long. Standing on a padded mat is a great way to improve the comfort and duration of your standing efforts. You'll know when it's time to transition to sitting over the course of the day, so pay attention, stay comfortable, and stay committed to the effort.

If you work for a large company with a facilities support staff, request standup adaptations such as a higher shelf on which to rest your computer. Or, if you decide to take matters into your own hands and make your own simple standup environment, all you need are a couple reams of paper, shipping boxes, or a footstool to elevate your keyboard and monitor. (Consider getting assistance to make sure your setup is safe and ergonomically optimum.) Once you become a convert, you can order a sophisticated standup workstation. But before you buy anything, test out different workstation heights. Measure the one that works best, and keep that measurement handy when you're shopping or building. For great ideas, check out the possibilities at Ergo Desktop at ErgoDesktop.com and Stand'nSitWorkstation at StandinGoodHealth.com.

SECTION SUMMARY

Stay in Touch: Touch is the most primitive of the senses, and in traditional societies it plays an extensive role. We are hardwired for neurochemical rewards from the touch we share with others, strengthening pair bonds and parent-child connections. Touch is a silent, potent language providing comfort and healing. And we don't call them pets for nothing; touching animals can provide the same benefits. Hugs, pats, hand-holding, cuddles, and massage serve us healthy helpings of that all-important oxytocin.

Go Barefoot: The elevated heel support found in most shoes impedes our natural gait and can cause lower extremity pain and injury, skew postural alignment, and compromise correct form during activity. Evolution aligned our leg contour, hip placement, and spinal structure for barefoot travel. A radical idea, perhaps, but going shoeless can improve your coordination, agility, balance, posture, and gait. Transition slowly to allow your feet and legs to adapt properly. When it isn't feasible to go totally barefoot, wear minimalist footwear such as flip-flops or Vibram FiveFingers.

Power of Posture: The spinal cord is essentially a high-bandwidth system for the transfer of information between nerves, organs, and other parts of our anatomy. Misalignments of the spine constrict nerve pathways and thus create pain. Esther Gokhale and other posture experts believe the ideal spine shape is a J-shaped spine, not the S-curved spine promoted by conventional medicine. The bones of a J-shaped spine are stacked in a straight line from the neck down through the lower back. One of the most common forms of bad posture is when the head leans forward instead of extending straight up from the shoulders. And don't forget proper potty posture. We are built to squat, but the "comfort" of modern sit-down toilets inhibits our ability to fully evacuate the bowels, increasing the risk of serious health conditions.

Made to Move: When you move, you kick hormones into gear with fat- and calorie-burning benefits. Stand-up desks or workstations, or homemade adaptations, allow you to stand comfortably without bending or straining. Make a concerted effort to engage in regular, comfortably paced aerobic workouts, as well as assorted general efforts to move more in daily life. Pay particular attention to taking brief movement breaks to counter prolonged periods of sitting or static standing.

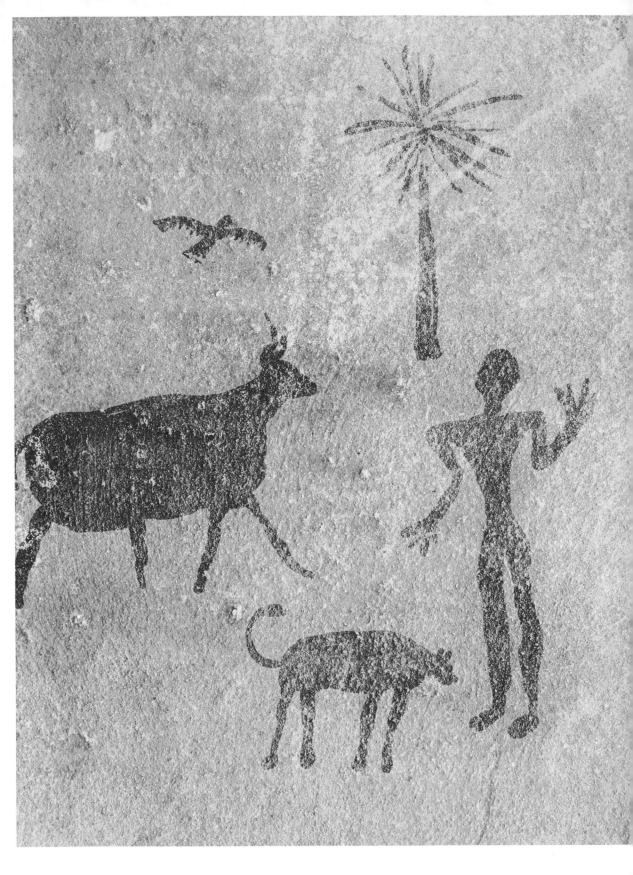

THE NATURE CONNECTION

TO OUR HUNTER-GATHERER GENES, the modern-day world looks, sounds, and feels a lot like living on another planet. Buildings and high-rises block or distort our view of the horizon and expansive sky, compromising the most simple and powerful perspective we have of our physical relationship to the Earth. Horns, sirens, and machines batter our aural faculties with a never-ending stream of noise. Neon signs and monster-sized billboards compete aggressively and incessantly for our attention without our permission. Traffic jams, long lines, interruptions, distractions, and big egos are woven into daily life in such a pervasive manner that we don't even realize the piece—or rather the peace—that's missing from our lives. In this section, we will look at ways to reconnect to the natural environs from which we evolved, finding, at last, peace and balance among the madness.

In all things of nature there is something of the marvelous.

ARISTOTLE

THE WILD WITHIN

OUR GENES PREDISPOSE US to prefer the sights, smells, sounds, and sensations of the wide-open savanna, amid the chirping of birds, the feel of rain, and the scent of vegetation. Indeed, our ancestors lived an earthy and sensual existence, seamlessly part of the natural world in ways that elude us now. Imagine what it must have been like to be surrounded by animal calls, noting the movement patterns in a river, perceiving the subtle clues or smells that arise while on the lookout for lurking predators. What thoughts must have run through our ancestors' minds while staring at the star-filled night sky? We've abandoned an essential source of our humanity and neglected a vital instinct that holds more sway over our wellbeing than we might think.

However transcendental a force we claim human intelligence is, we are still beings of the wild. True, our species developed a unique and powerful ability to manipulate the natural world. But to deny or dismiss nature's place in our otherwise high-tech lives is naïve and perilous to our psychological and physical health. As ecopsychiatrist Anthony Stevens suggests, wilderness is more than just an external "place." Nature is that genetic aspect of ourselves that spatially occupies every body and every cell.[1]

We often fail to understand or foster this attachment. With the perpetual march of technological progress and deepening isolation of urbanization, nature is more remote than ever in our lives. Yet another example of what once was abundant now is scarce. When we build our lives so withdrawn from the wild and consider our status so remote from its animal inhabitants, it can be difficult to perceive our innate belonging in the natural world.

Yet, the nagging bit of our evolutionary selves remains—those stubborn vestiges of past millennia, original instincts operating from the age-old hunter-gatherer framework. Human ingenuity knows no bounds. Human genes, however, do. We still exist enmeshed in the natural world both physiologically and psychologically. However fulfilled or unfulfilled these expectations are for us, our biological selves were designed to participate within the natural world. In rediscovering the wild, we emancipate our own true nature.

A SENSUAL WORLD

What characterizes our mindset in nature, that involuntary bottom-up attention that has the power to reset us mentally? The key is in the senses. You may notice as you spend more time in nature that your involuntary awareness takes over, and your senses become heightened. Sounds are quieter but more subtly layered. Your sight is more expansive. Your sense of touch, finer. Your sense of smell, more acute. Surrounded by nature, your perception reorients to its default setting. Instinctively, you know this and have likely experienced it. Whenever you step outside your commotion-filled asphalt environment and truly inhabit a wild space, you're more relaxed but sharply aware.

Think of the textures and sensations you might encounter while clearing brush for a campsite or hopping along boulders to reach a water source. What sort of biofeedback might you encounter from the environment? Rough, prickly, sharp, slick, porous? A lot more interesting, don't you think, than walking on cement in your clunky shoes from the parking lot to

YOU ARE HARDWIRED to encounter the sights, sounds, scents, and sensations found in nature.

MODERN DISCONNECT: the din of the city and sterile indoor environments.

PRIMAL CONNECTION: nature immersion.

> **" Our ability to hear predators and interpret the auditory cues of our environment was perhaps the most crucial to our ancestors' survival. "**

the elevator, then sitting at a desk amidst entirely artificial objects that are so smoothed out and shaped that your tactile faculties begin to atrophy?

Of all our senses, one of the most complex and fundamental is our sense of hearing. Turns out we're intended to be an aurally oriented species. Our ability to hear predators and interpret the auditory cues of our environment was perhaps the most crucial to our ancestors' survival. Today, instead of encountering the original sound track of our evolutionary roots—low-decibel, natural sounds such as birds chirping, distant animal cries, running water, the rustle of leaves in the wind, and so forth—we're faced with an orgy of noise consisting of traffic, sirens, ringtones, honking horns, jet planes, police helicopters, lawn mowers and, worst of the lot—leaf blowers! Yet for the amount of noise we take in, we are, according to some experts, aurally deficient. We're starved for those subtle layers of natural sounds our brains evolved to perceive and process. As George Prochnik, author of *Pursuit of Silence: Listening for Meaning in a World of Noise*, explains, it's like we stuff ourselves with junk-food noise but still hunger for the sound that truly nourishes us.

It gets worse: a 2012 study, published in the *Journal of Neuroscience*, revealed that sounds stimulate the amygdala, the part of the brain that processes emotions.[2] It turns out that our perception of unpleasant sounds like electric drills and the squeal of braking tires (or most anything in the frequency range of 2,000 to 5,000 Hz) is heightened compared to soothing sounds such as bubbling water or invigorating sounds like the clapping of hands. Though natural sounds are less affecting on our emotions than unpleasant ones, they do have a strong influence on our wellbeing, countering stress and urban noise, making us more relaxed and aware, and, according to one study, helping to manage acute illness and pain.[3]

As for our sense of smell, few synthetic scents, intense as they can be, are capable of synchronizing with our other senses quite the way natural aromas do. Think of the delicate scents you encounter during a walk, let's say after a rainfall (ozone), or through a deciduous forest (musty), or on the beach and you experience a gust of sea breeze (briny). Perhaps in the moment you recall a long-ago memory. Or you create a new one. This would be no accident: the olfactory nerve in the brain is separated by only three synapses from the hippocampus and two synapses from the amygdala, which are respectively responsible for processing long-term and emotional memory.

So, does it make sense that as we pay attention to the more subtle nuances from our environment, we simultaneously expand our intelligence? Darn right, it does! "Our brains are able to make use of subtler and subtler stimuli, to be inventive and create new connections, possibilities, and solutions," writes psychologist and brain-based healing expert Anat Baniel in *Move into Life: The Nine Essentials for Lifelong Vitality*. "This ability to feel finer and finer differences is at the heart of what we call intuition."

RESTORING THE HARDWARE

Our primal brains are hardwired to process every last bit of disruptive sensory input that we face, ready to alarm us to either fight or flee. Resolving to ignore billboards, Zen out on your subway ride, or filter out honking horns cannot completely override this genetic coding. Even if you love the excitement that the big city has to offer, you simply cannot change the fact that the overstimulation it provides taxes the brain's inhibitory attention far beyond what it has evolved to withstand. You may argue that you truly love the din of the city or the frenzied crowd at the ball game or rock concert. But when you are continually stressed in such a manner, you lose your ability to focus on a given task for any prolonged period of time.

Known as *directed attention fatigue*, this neurological disorder is a wholly modern affliction. The good news is that exposure to nature reverses its effects. Your perception—that is, your involuntary attention—amid natural surroundings creates a calm mental picture, partly because sounds in nature typically carry at lower decibels and are more predictable than the random, jolting stimuli you are forced to deal with in most urban environments. Compare the sounds of breaking waves to honking horns, for example. The same holds true with vision. Your sight is more expansive as you alternately focus on close and distant objects. Contrast this with staring at the two dimensions of a computer screen thirty inches from your face all day!

Nature indeed produces therapeutic effects on us. Since the 1960s, environmental psychologists Rachel and Stephen Kaplan have become well known for their attention restoration theory, which states that if we are to flourish as humans—and preserve the mental and physical health that the hustle and bustle of civilized life jeopardizes—we require frequent exposure to tranquil, natural settings.

Among the most compelling research that supports this theory is that of "forest therapy," currently practiced in Japan. Studies there show that time in a wooded setting unleashes a powerful cascade of hormonal and cellular responses. Salivary cortisol, a marker for stress, for example, dropped an average of 13.4 percent when subjects simply looked at a forest setting for twenty minutes.[4] Pulse rate, blood pressure, and activity on the sympathetic (fight-or-flight) nervous system decreased as well. Even more remarkable is the significant— and lasting—impact on so-called "natural killer" cells (NK cells), powerful lymphocytes known to fight off infection and attack cancer growth. A longer three-day trip in the forest with daily walks resulted in a 50 percent rise in NK activity as well as an increase in the number of NK cells! What's perhaps most surprising is this: subjects who participated in this series of forest-bathing trips showed immune NK benefits that lasted more than a month.[5] As a result of these studies, government entities in Japan are partnering with the medical industry to hold free health checkups at park areas and to create designations for "official" forest therapy sites. Finally, more companies are opting to include forest therapy in health care plans.

Water restores your brain and body, too. Consider this passage from a 2011 article in *Outside* magazine featuring Michael Merzenich, a neuroscience professor at University of California, San Francisco and one of the foremost authorities on neuro-plasticity.

> Our attraction to the ocean may derive from its lack of physical markers. On land, we are constantly mapping our environment in our minds so we can pick out dangers (snake!) amid landmarks (tree, bush, rock). Looking over a calm sea is akin to closing our eyes. And when something does emerge on the surface, it captivates us.[6]

Indeed, there's nothing more relaxing as looking at or being in a body of water. Whether it's an ocean, a lake, a small river, we're quite simply transfixed. We easily let go of whatever ails or distracts us.

If you actually enter the water, things get even better. The mere act of floating produces a calming feeling by activating the parasympathetic nervous system (PSN), which is responsible for stimulating rest and digestion when the body is at rest. When you float, you reduce your body weight by nearly 90 percent, providing therapeutic benefits to your joints and muscles. Submerge yourself under the water, and you become totally present in the moment and enter a deeper dimension of sensory fascination. (An effect surely intensified by not having any air to breathe!) Even the high-intensity sport of surfing provides relaxation to the mind and body that transcends the sport into everyday life. Philippe Goldin, a clinical psychologist and a neuroscientist at Stanford University, notes that surfers, thanks to their proximity to the water, are able to experience reflective, meditation-like downtime between wave sets, helping them balance the fight-or-flight reaction to approaching swells.[7] The US Marine Corps has also recognized

FEET ON THE GROUND

The concept of "earthing," also known as grounding, suggests that with the advent of shoes, houses, flooring, and elevated beds, we've largely eliminated direct bodily contact to the inherent electrical field of the earth. There's actually some sound science behind it. Thermography images and blood samples from patients who responded poorly to conventional medications and therapies revealed a surprising reduction in inflammation and improved blood viscosity after thirty minutes of earthing—sitting, walking, or standing on conductive surfaces such as grass, sand, and dirt.[10] (Bear in mind, grounding does not work on wood, asphalt, or vinyl surfaces.) Others report reduced physical pain and emotional stress.[11] Research shows that earthing can encourage a better night's sleep, moderate nighttime cortisol levels, and enhance circadian synchronization.[12] See if you can go barefoot, connected to the ground when you go about your endeavors. It's clear that many of us have heavily, or almost entirely, neglected direct contact to the earth in daily life and can likely benefit from not only the electrical connection, but the ancillary benefits of making the effort.

these benefits, using "surf therapy" as a therapeutic intervention for sufferers of post-traumatic stress disorder. Of course, the negative ions that result from the crashing waves likely have a profound effect as well.

THE POWER OF NEGATIVE IONS

Negative ions (good stuff, as we'll learn shortly) generally appear in natural settings in greater numbers than positive ions (bad stuff, despite their name). But what exactly are ions? They are atoms or molecules in which the number of electrons is different from the number of protons. If an ion is negatively charged, it has more electrons than protons. If it is positively charged, it has more protons than electrons.

We find an abundance of negative ions wherever air molecules are split by solar radiation, wind, and water. That's great news for us! These tiny, highly reactive, molecular fragments energize your body at the cellular level. They help increase the flow of oxygen to the brain, resulting in higher alertness, decreased drowsiness, and more mental energy.

Think of the times you've experienced their effects: near breaking ocean waves, a waterfall, or a sunny, windy, mountain area. These represent the ultimate in negative ion experiences—we're talking about inhaling air enriched with tens of thousands of negative ions per cubic centimeter.

By comparison, fresh air in the countryside might rate 4,000 per cubic centimeter, a high-traffic urban area might contain less than a hundred per cubic centimeter, and a stagnant home or office might measure in the dozens or even zero! And while not as impressive as getting misted on the observation deck at Niagara Falls, your shower is another handy way to get an energizing dose of negative ions. Plants also produce negative ions, especially when exposed to intense light during photosynthesis.

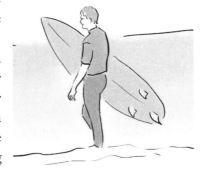

Now for the rub: positive ions collect in pollution and soot, recirculated indoor air, or any enclosed space such as a car, train, office, or home. Positive ions have an adverse effect on your body. They trap and neutralize negative ions, robbing the air of its vitality and promoting fatigue and assorted health problems. Electrical appliances such as computers and televisions also generate positive ions, as do high-voltage power lines.

Studies with NASA astronauts suggest that ion imbalance can promote fatigue, bone loss, compromised sleep cycles, and overactive adrenal glands, which leads to burnout and compromised immune function.[8] Other studies suggest excess positive ions and insufficient negative ions can result in anxiety, depression, electrolyte imbalances, systemic inflammation, emotional disturbances, and diminished cardiovascular and brain function.[9]

Since ions are electrical, the effects of natural and artificial ionization are identical. This is good news for your home and office, because you can purchase a negative ion generator for as little as fifty dollars at a good office supply or

WATER THERAPY

Cold-water immersion is a great example of hormesis—a brief, positive, natural stressor. Nearly every morning I experience an hormetic response when I plunge into cold water for a minute or two in my unheated swimming pool, which usually stands around 68 degrees in the summer and the low 50s in the winter, and then I air-dry in the sun. During a hormetic response, your brain signals your adrenals to release the stress hormone cortisol. Such responses, as previously mentioned, are undesirable with long-term, chronic exposure. But short-term exposure leaves you with a sense of eustress (good stress that is within or just slightly outside your comfort zone) as your body attempts to return to homeostasis.

Research confirms that short bouts of cold-water immersion benefits immune function and muscle recovery.[15] While Cold Thermogenesis (CT), a prolonged exposure to cold water for the purpose of accelerating fat burning, is a hot topic in Evolutionary Health circles these days, I recommend briefer exposure times (if you're getting cold, time to get out!) to enjoy the benefits immune and invigoration benefit without the risks of chronic stress. However, there is evidence that cold immersion enhances recovery from intense training sessions, so go ahead and soak your legs in an icy stream after a hard run for a few minutes!

home electronics store. I recommend a combination deionizer/HEPA machine that will remove both particulate matter (pollen, dust, mold) and noxious gases (smoke, toxic auto, and industry emissions).

EXERCISE YOUR SENSES

Next time you have a free hour, head outdoors. Find a park bench, a quiet place in your yard, a drive out to a local water source, the beach, a lake, or a pond. Quiet your mind, engage your senses, and be fully aware of your surroundings. Allow your eyes to soak in the scenery. Take notice of the colors and movements around you. Listen for subtleties: Do you hear birds chirping? Water running? Maybe the wind passing through the leaves? Pick up a leaf, feel its contoured details, and open up to textures you've not noticed before. Employ your sense of smell. Can you identify anything interesting in the air, maybe a distinct foliage, humidity, or animal life? After a few minutes of processing, think about the contrast between what you have just experienced and the in-your-face stimulation of a phone, computer, television, or busy office. Here's a list of some other easy options that can help you exercise your senses and reconnect with nature.

Grab a handful of soil. Smell it and crumble it between your fingers.
Watch the clouds for five minutes.
Create a small sandbox. Put your feet in and wiggle your toes.
Go barefoot outdoors. Every day, and yes, even in winter.
Set up a bird feeder outside your window. Enjoy the sense of community.
Find a stream. Ditch the shoes and socks and step in.
Go outside. Find something different every day to smell.
Drop absolutely everything. Go outside and listen.
Bring your book outside. Do a little reading amidst nature.
Stop to appreciate the moon. Full or otherwise.
Pick a favorite tree. It can be in your yard, your neighborhood, or near your work site. Notice how it changes with the seasons.
Be in full contact with the earth. Lie on the grass. Roll down a hill. Jump off a berm.
Handle the vegetation. Feel the leaves and bark of every tree in your yard, the flowers in your pots, a patch of wild grasses.

I cannot have a spiritual center without having a
geographical one; I cannot live a grounded life without
being grounded in a place.

Scott Russell Sanders

RECLAIMING THE OUTDOORS

In his time, set against the backdrop of the Industrial Revolution, Henry David Thoreau's notion that humans are an extension of nature—rather than rulers of it—was considered quite radical. No one, he believed, ought to feel lonely in the company of the outdoors. We can find company in a dandelion, a horsefly, even Walden Pond itself. The point is, we are of nature, not separate from it. Yet a century and a half after penning his classic work, even as we make strides to undo the grit and grime of industry and return to a greener planet, this simple truth still eludes many of us.

If you can't swing living in a remote cabin and doing nothing but observing nature from dawn till noon, as Thoreau was wont to do, you can certainly look at ways to move more elements of your life outdoors. Try taking your coffee breaks and lunch breaks outside. If you have kids, exercise some vigilance against the Digital Age by balancing their screen time with outdoor playtime. Maybe even spend a night outside sleeping under the stars.

My wife, Carrie, and I enjoy doing just that very thing when weather permits. It's hardly a rugged wilderness experience with the patio sliding door a few paces away. But it's a refreshing change of pace, gazing at the stars, the clouds, the moon. Try it yourself at home. Soak in the panorama and see if your peripheral vision picks up a shooting star. Even just fifteen or twenty minutes under the night sky can be enough to clear your head.

If you aren't the type who can sit still and just be, how about sampling the amazing mobile astronomy technology that's available today? Apps such as Google Sky (Android platform) and Star Walk (for Apple's iOS) allow you to point your device toward the sky and instantly map planets, moons, asteroids, comets, stars, and constellations. Or check out a local astronomy group (search online or at your local community college), and avail yourself of a world of experts with powerful telescopes and organized outings.

Get creative, take full advantage of the temperate seasons, and head out to the desert or mountains for an overnight camping trip. At the very least, create an inviting area to relax, work, or eat in your yard, on your porch, or on your balcony. Whether you favor yoga, meditation, stretching, or body resistance exercises, find a place to do them outdoors to maximize the overall benefits. And do make it a social event by encouraging others to participate.

As for don'ts: don't be a weather wimp! Far too many folks balk at outdoor activity unless the weather du jour falls within a few degrees of their climate-controlled environs. Cold outside? Slap on a hat and coat and go out in nature. If it's hot, don a cap (or not) and appreciate the energy and warmth of the sun's rays hitting your skin. The point is, leave the excuses and rationalizations behind and get out there. I'm betting you'll feel invigorated by the experience.

If you dwell in an urban center and have ready-made excuses for neglecting nature, do a retake. Virtually every urban center has its own nature escapes just a short distance away—even if it's just a small park or playground. Look into nearby hiking and biking trails. If you're into organized outings, look into joining a club like the Audubon Society, Sierra Club, or local Nature Conservancy.

At home, take a cue from nature and add natural elements such as wood, stone, or even metal, and natural light. Live plants especially make quick and inexpensive additions. They not only look great, but act as natural air scrubbers by removing much of the CO^2 from the air and filtering out Volatile Organic Compounds (VOCs) such as trichloroethylene, benzene, and formaldehyde, which are commonly found in paints, varnishes, building materials, and paper and personal hygiene products. The best type of plant is one officially categorized as "houseplant." They evolved to flourish under the canopy of large trees, so they do well indoors.

Some of the houseplants singled out in NASA's 1989 Clean Air Study are areca palm (great general purifier), bamboo (acts as natural humidifier), peace lily (removes mold spores), gerbera daisy (absorbs carbon dioxide—great for bedrooms to improve overnight oxygen absorption), snake plant (absorbs nitrogen oxides), and spider plant (removes carbon monoxide). Aloe plants are also great, pulling double duty as an air scrubber and powerful skin-healing gel.

Artwork and photos that depict nature provide nearly the same positive effect on our psyches as the real thing. Same goes for piped-in natural sounds. So be sure to include those in your living environment as well, especially if your home environment is lacking in other natural features. In one 2008 study, subjects had access to either windows covered with curtains or high-definition plasma TVs (made to look like windows) depicting realistic nature scenes. The folks who saw the technological nature had improved psychological wellbeing, cognitive functioning, and a sense of "connection to the natural world," while folks who saw the covered windows did not.[13]

One of my favorite indoor features is a saltwater fish tank, which can provide countless hours of peace and tranquility. You may also wish to open your home to pet birds, cats, or reptiles. But there is perhaps no better companion for reclaiming the outdoors than with man's best friend.

Studies of dog-human interactions confirm the biological benefits, reporting increased levels of the hormone oxytocin, the so-called "love hormone" (not to be confused with the commonly abused painkiller oxycontin). After positive social interactions, your body releases oxytocin, promoting feelings of contentment, empathy, strengthened social bonding, and reduced fear and anxiety.

While evidence suggests the domestication of dogs dates back some thirty thousand years, the interaction between wolves and early humans goes back nearly one hundred thousand years. One theory holds that canines domesticated themselves,[14] learning quickly that wherever man went, bones and scraps would surely follow. Having a dog offers you to a display of primal behavior all day long, from the succession of

YOU ARE HARDWIRED *to thrive in open spaces, interacting with nature.*

MODERN DISCONNECT: *spending large amounts of time in enclosed spaces such as cars, trains, stores, home, and office.*

PRIMAL CONNECTION: *Move elements of indoor life outdoors; simulate nature sights and sounds.*

> **"Artwork and photos that depict nature provide nearly the same positive effect on our psyches as the real thing."**

power naps, to the immediate spring to attention for the life-or-death matter of a random squirrel invading your buddy's territory.

The next time your dog bravely wards off a furry intruder or proudly drops a souvenir mouse or bird catch on the front porch or kitchen floor, take a moment to savor natural animal instincts in action. And this is just backyard stuff I'm talking about. Get your dog out for a proper hike in the wilderness, and watch him bound up a near-vertical incline, muzzle into every nook and cranny along the trail, and leap half-madly into any and all bodies of water. Maybe you can follow suit? If a dog can't get you in touch with your inner beast, I dare say nothing can. Just be sure to bring enough blankets to cover the entire backseat of the car for the ride home!

If for some reason your living situation does not allow you to add a canine to your home life, look into volunteering at your local animal shelter or animal rescue. They are always looking for animal lovers to spend quality time petting and visiting with their broods. To follow are a few additional ideas to help you reclaim the outdoors. Let your imagination run free and expand on these suggestions with more of your own:

Attract critters. Plant flowers that attract butterflies. If you live on the West Coast, be sure to catch the bi-annual migration of the Monarch butterflies between Canada and Baja California. Or pick up a bag of ladybugs for the garden—a natural predator to unwelcome pests.

Perform dawn patrol. Enjoy your morning coffee with the sunrise. Better yet, venture out for a hike or walk around the block at dawn. It almost always turns into a memorable experience.

Observe and record. Grab a guidebook and a pair of binoculars and become a bird watcher or hobby botanist. Take up nature photography and travel in search of breathtaking scenery and wildlife. Or grab a field bag and collect interesting artifacts. Get into polishing stones or refinishing driftwood. Savor the fun of collecting natural souvenirs, but always be respectful to not disturb the natural environment.

Step into liquid. I lean more to the serenity of standup paddling myself, but any activity involving water promotes a strong and inherent nature connection. Choose from high-adrenaline stuff (surfing, wakesurfing, kitesurfing, waterskiing, wakeboarding), paddle activities (kayak, canoe, standup paddling), underwater endeavors (snorkeling, SCUBA, freediving), or something completely mellow such as floating down a river in an inner tube.

Dine al fresco. Take your meals outside when you can. This is especially fun in groups. Outdoor gatherings provide a more relaxed, mellow vibe and are made especially fun when an outdoor movie screening is included. Just set up an LCD projector hitting a portable screen or white sheet draped on an outdoor wall.

Be a kid again. Puddle stomp, pick in-season fruit, walk on the beach, hike up to the water tower, or fly a kite in the park. What did you love doing outdoors when you were a youngster? What the heck happened? Weave those things back into your life one by one.

SCOPING YOUR HABITAT

Reconnecting with the wild requires a deep familiarity with the land. As George B. Silberbauer puts it in *Hunter and Habitat in the Central Kalahari Desert*, no one should be a stranger to a place he or she occupies for any length of time. We evolved identifying with our habitat, even if it was a considerably vast area of hunting and gathering potential. Such connections to the land are still evidenced today in societies of indigenous people.

The Australian Aborigines, for example, have navigated their terrain through the use of *songlines* for forty thousand years. These songs, or vocal maps, are sung in specific sequences containing lyrics, rhythms, and melodies that correspond to the land's geographical features. Going to a specific watering hole, for instance, might require singing a particular songline about a watering hole sixteen times until you reach the marker. Once there, the songline changes en route to the next marker on the path, a cave, perhaps, and is sung the appropriate number of times until reaching the cave. Some songlines are known to spread hundreds of kilometers across the Australian interior. The songlines pass through regions and groups of widely disparate tribal cultures, adapting into other languages. (There are over a hundred dialects among the Aboriginal peoples). This might read as a charming anecdote for those of us with handheld GPS navigation apps, but for our primal ancestors, and traditional societies like the indigenous Australians, intimate knowledge of terrain was, and still is, a matter of survival.

> ## You connect with your habitat by acting within it, moving within it, and engaging your senses and imagination.

This obligation to claim one's habitat was so powerful in primal life that all of culture reflected and celebrated an attachment to the land. In his memoirs of living with traditional communities, anthropologist Wade Davis elaborates: "Mythology infuses land and life with meaning, encoding expectations and behaviors essential to survival in the forest, anchoring each community ... to a profound spirit of place."[16]

Who our ancestors were and how they defined themselves was inextricable from their terrain. Few of us have totemic associations connecting ancestry to animals or spirits anymore, but the essential truth of connection to your habitat lingers. Those of us who still live in the towns and countryside of our family's previous generations can perhaps identify with this concept more easily. The land is part of your story—it's part of you. But no matter how well you think you know the woods behind your house, the garden out back, the lake down the street, or the local hiking trails, there's always potential for more subtle, ongoing discovery.

Sometimes, the connection you have to your home base doesn't hit you until you return from a hiatus. As writer Richard Louv suggests, travel has the power to astound you with the sheer magnitude and diversity of the world and to help you perceive gratefully the character and life of your own terrain.[17] You return home to a sense of belonging—not just to your house and possessions, but also to your habitat. And what if you have been permanently or semipermanently uprooted, say, for job opportunities or some other reason? There are still many ways to live reciprocally and meaningfully in an unfamiliar land. Wherever you are, the land calls upon you to invest is a little time, interest, and attention.

Seek out the historical areas of any city, and you'll likely find natural monuments such as the oldest trees, largest ponds, riverfronts, or the other landscape features that shaped the original urban layout. Likewise, there are little-known preserve areas, bike trails, architectural points of interest, community gardens, and, of course, alternate routes to get you where you want to go. Nothing delights me more than discovering a clever shortcut to bypass a cluttered major intersection!

You connect with your habitat by acting within it, moving within it, and engaging your senses and imagination. No GPS required, just set foot out your door, and see where the landscape of people, activity, and architecture leads you. If you are intent on your walk, you can't help but exercise Habit #4: be present. Your inner dialogue should sound a little like this: "Look at that leaf; it's shaped like an elephant's ear." "Look at that rust spot on that gate." "There's a ceramic turtle on the lawn over there I never noticed before." "There's a new cobweb under that mailbox." There are easily a thousand new things you could notice about your surroundings if you try. But challenge yourself to pick at least twenty. This is not at all unlike what our ancestors did, who had to pick up on every available clue and know everything there was to know about a trail back to their home camp.

Take this time also to appreciate contemplative solitude or act on opportunities to make new acquaintances. Lose yourself for an afternoon meandering through a familiar place and looking at it from a new vantage point. Once you do, you'll never see it quite the same way again.

Consider kicking your habitat adventures up a notch and actually record what you encounter over

YOU ARE HARDWIRED *to be intimately attuned to and familiar with your surroundings.*

MODERN DISCONNECT: *navigating your terrain by car and GPS while your focus is someplace else.*

PRIMAL CONNECTION: *explore your home terrain on foot.*

a month, a season, a year—or more. Think of it as your personal *Walden*. Choose a medium such as photography, video, or journaling, and record your neighborhood observations. Decipher patterns in the area's wildlife. A small lake in the middle of a large city can be host to frogs, turtles, cranes, geese, and all sorts of other creatures. Even a quiet street can have its share of birds and gardens. Likewise, take note of the human cast of characters you regularly encounter while exploring your habitat—the man who commutes by cross-country skiing on winter evenings, the two older women who walk arm-in-arm down the street speaking a foreign language, the child who sits in an ornamental tree with a book after school each day. You'll note what the neighborhood looks and feels like after a snowstorm, with the changing of the leaves, or during a drizzly day. The more aware you are of your surroundings, the more you'll discover the extraordinary.

*To forget how to dig the earth and
to tend the soil is to forget ourselves.*

MAHATMA GANDHI

PLAY DIRTY

FOR 2.5 MILLION YEARS, our ancestors consumed food that was encrusted with bits of dirt teeming with germs and other microbes. What we would regard as filth today is in fact how our ancestors populated and repopulated their guts with beneficial bacteria. It's only within the last century that we've gone overboard with sanitizing our environment. Again, what was once abundant—constant interaction with dirt, germs, natural water sources, and all sorts of other organic matter teeming with bacteria—is now relatively scarce. And our immune systems suffer accordingly.

Our immune systems are made up of a complex army of leukocytes, what we commonly refer to as white blood cells, which are of several types, each specializing in a certain set of duties. They circulate through the bloodstream, constantly on the lookout for invaders, ready to attack when necessary. In defending our bodies, their mission is to show up on two fronts: one known as the *innate* immune system and the other as the *adaptive* immune system. The innate system responds automatically to routine security breaches, such as a bee sting or scraped knee. Macrophages, neutrophils, natural killer cells (NK cells), and complement proteins rush to the scene of the invasion like microscopic RoboCops to gobble up and dispose of damaged tissue. The result is the familiar

> **Over the course of evolution, _Homo sapiens_ have come to host some sixty trillion microbes of beneficial bacteria, weighing as much as six pounds!**

swelling of an injured area—all part of the master plan to contain, and then rid your body of undesirables and return you quickly and smoothly to homeostasis.

The adaptive immune system is just as stealthy. It learns through exposure and experience, and almost always recognizes the infectious agents it has previously encountered. It sends in troops of B cells (from your bone marrow) and T cells (from your thymus organ, located in the center of your chest), which multiply like crazy and destroy the offending organism. These attacks are swift, efficient, and elegantly coordinated. What's more, the adaptive immune system, like a hard-boiled five-star general, has a keen memory for the intimate details of each battle fought. At any given moment—for the rest of your life—it stands ready to implement a winning strategy should the same foreign microorganism return.

But here's the thing: your immune system, though it operates as a germ-killing machine protecting the fort, is not self-contained. It behaves more like a peacekeeping envoy within your bacteria-laden environment. That is to say, we're meant to live side by side among most germs quite harmoniously. Over the course of evolution, _Homo sapiens_ have come to host some sixty trillion microbes of beneficial bacteria, weighing as much as six pounds! Your particular microbe composition is unique and ever-changing, the better to continually assist with optimal digestion, immune function, and crowding out all that harmful bacteria you encounter at home, at work, on the subway, and from every hand you shake or doorknob you touch. Even if you're a clean freak who just stepped out of a long, hot, scrubby shower, your body immediately attracts hordes of harmful bacteria, viruses, fungi, and protozoa. Your resident healthy bacteria usually make short work of these invading interlopers before they can cause any problems.

Before the twentieth century, humans did not experience a highly sanitized existence. That we live in one today is not such a bad thing either. Since the

1860s, with basic sanitation practices that includes the simple act of hand washing, infection risks in childbirth and death during major surgery has been greatly neutralized. Food- and water-borne illnesses are extremely rare today, too. However, germ-free living (not to mention the plastics, chemicals, and environmental toxins that are part of the whole sanitizing-of-society deal) remains a shock to our primal genes. Like a benchwarmer on the basketball team, if your immune system doesn't see enough action, it's difficult for it to perform when it is called to play.

Increases in allergies, asthma, autism, obesity, type 1 diabetes, mood disorders, multiple sclerosis, inflammatory bowel disease, and other conditions related to systemic inflammation or autoimmune dysfunction are partially blamed on our lack of exposure to dirt! Referred to as the hygiene hypothesis, it is the notion that we are becoming *too* clean, evidenced by an increase in the aforementioned conditions only in countries that are the *most* developed and sanitized. Lower rates of immune disturbances are seen in families with pets (another good reason to hang with man's best friend!), families living on farms, and among the youngest siblings in large families, presumably due to increased exposure to germs from animals, and in busy households with parents relaxing their hygiene standards with successive kids. (Can you say, "five-second rule?")

Exposure to actual soil, as well as the organic carrots you bring home from the farmers market, or the mouthful of seawater inhaled while playing in the surf are especially critical for the proper development of a child's immature immune system. Each invading microbe-versus-healthy bacterium event that occurs daily in a child's body represents a valuable home-school lesson for her immune system. Toddlers, when they escape the range of a helicopter parent, are inclined to lick or swallow varied cuisine such as dried horse poop, leftover dog food, Play-Doh, pill bugs, you name it. One recent magazine article mentioned the contents of a cremation urn knocked over by a toddler!

Go ahead and cringe, but toddlers are expressing a critical primal instinct with their oral fixations.

YOU ARE HARDWIRED *to come in contact with germs and microbes without adverse effects.*

MODERN DISCONNECT: *overly sanitizing yourself and your environments.*

PRIMAL CONNECTION: *get dirty and boost immune function in the process.*

The ingestion of fill-in-the-blank organic matter introduces a number of bacteria and viruses that spur the development of their immature systems. The kid with a dirty mouth isn't increasing his chances of getting sick— he's actually giving his immune system practice in figuring out what's benign and what's dangerous. He's establishing a critical baseline that will influence his immune response throughout his lifetime. Note that I'm talking about exposure to organic matter here. I do not advocate exposing yourself or your child to toxic chemicals, intentional exposure to sneezing classmates, raw hamburger meat, or inorganic, solid objects like marbles and coins that present a choking threat. What I'm talking about instead is watching your kid wipe his nose, pet his dog, wipe the railing on the park slide, then stick his fingers in his mouth … and you not freaking out and saturating his entire upper body with antibacterial wipes!

Yes, loosening your obsessive hygiene standards may result in assorted illnesses and infections, but this is all part of the training process. Each time you battle a bug, you improve the communication and fighting skills of your immune system to succeed in future battles. The most critical time of the immune system maturation process is during infancy, because there is a narrow window of opportunity during which human T cells can develop optimally and offer lifelong protection.

Vigorous efforts to protect yourself and your family from coming in contact with organic matter essentially messes around with the intricate interaction between man and germ, a relationship that has been with us from the very beginning. Such interferences make it difficult for your body to discern friend from foe. It can become hyperactive and disoriented, misfiring repeatedly against harmless stuff such as seasonal pollen and grass. Your body may even experience a civil war of sorts, with a flawed immune system inclined to turn upon itself, which is what happens in cases of autoimmune disorders.

Ditch any soap, wipe, or spray in your house that has antibacterial properties *right now!* Is your inner clean freak balking at the mere suggestion? Then just imagine, as you scrub your skin with powerful germ-killing agents, that you are eliminating billions of beneficial bacteria—basically stripping away your protective barrier—and clearing space for potential pathogens to take hold. Regular old soap and hot water is all you need to navigate modern life—really! Just sing the alphabet song while lathering your hands to ensure you actually achieve the intended result of clean hands. Practice safe handling with raw meat and other potentially contaminated foods, but know that everyday soap is effective even against salmonella and other big-shot microbes. And as a personal experiment, try a few baths and showers without the soap and shampoo. Use just a washcloth, and towel dry afterward.

What's more, modern society's obsession to eliminate germs and treat minor infections with powerful antibiotics has led to the formation of so-called superbugs that are resistant to typical sanitation efforts as well as commonly prescribed antibiotics.

Mary Ruebush, microbiology and immunology expert and author of *Why Dirt Is Good: Five Ways to Make Germs Your Friends*, offers an ominous observation about our modern germophobic habits: "Our desire to overwash, overbathe, and overmedicate our bodies causes changes in the normal populations of organisms (flora) that live in and on us …. The age of antibiotics—the miracle drugs such as penicillin that have saved countless lives—is perilously close to coming to an end. The blame lies squarely with us."

SAY HELLO TO FRIENDLY BACTERIA

Antibiotics do not discriminate—they kill the good with the bad. During and after your antibiotic treatment, be sure to take a probiotic supplement to repopulate the healthy flora in your intestinal tract. Eating plenty of raw vegetables, fresh fruits, and fermented foods (kefir, yogurt, kombucha, sauerkraut, kimchi) will also ensure that the beneficial bacteria flourish and predominate over the harmful. By the way, harmful bacteria feed off of sugar, refined grains, chemically altered fats, and other heavily processed foods. You may be deficient in healthy intestinal flora if you have recurring bad breath, cold sores, constipation, diarrhea, vaginal or yeast infections, or headaches. If so, make efforts to improve your diet, supplement with a probiotic, splash around in the mud, and dig around in the garden!

PRACTICAL TIPS TO GET DIRTY

When you dig, plant, and play in the soil, you receive a dose of potent bacteria that fine-tunes your immune system. Research shows that exposure to *Mycobacterium vaccae*, a bacterium commonly found in uncontaminated soil, stimulates the release of serotonin, which helps reduce anxiety, enhances your ability to develop new cognitive skills, and balances energy and emotions. The original source of this beneficial bacterium is none other than cow dung. (The word *vaccae* is derived from the Latin word for cow.) Interesting aside, perhaps, but on a more serious note, isn't it time to get over our tired conventional wisdom regarding sanitation, and reconnect with the enhanced mood, cognition, and immune function that dirt has to offer? Return to the days of our childhood love of mud, muck, and cowpies? Or, alternatively, any one of the suggestions to follow.

Creek stomping. Who needs an SUV? The Primal way is full body contact! Jump in the water—creek, brook, river, or stream—and cruise along on foot.

Indoor plants. Raise indoor plants or herb gardens. As you water, trim dead leaves, and re-pot or loosen compacted soil, you'll dose yourself amply with *M. vaccae* and her friendly cousins.

Lie down. While the tenth fairway or the elementary soccer field might look tempting, make an effort to discover earth that has not been manicured, such as a meadow, hillside, or beach. This will limit your risk of exposure to pesticides and other chemicals that are commonly used to create perfect, but unnatural, green areas.

Mud bath. Enthusiasts of mud and mineral immersion spas tout scientifically validated healing and cleansing powers for the skin and the circulatory system. It's also inherently relaxing to be immersed and suspended in a thick, warm mud bath. Studies suggest that mud baths possess anti-inflammatory properties, helping ease assorted aches and pains as well as painful skin conditions such as psoriasis and rosacea. You also absorb sodium, magnesium, potassium and other beneficial minerals into your skin.

Mud run. After a good rain, grab a dog, a kid, or a friend and go searching for the biggest, splashiest, muddiest puddles you can find. See how much of it you and your companions can accumulate on your body and clothing. These days, this is hardly a novel suggestion. Organized mud runs patterned after military boot camp obstacle courses are becoming quite the rage on the endurance events calendar. Look into one in your area to transform a routine road race into a diverse mental and physical challenge with immune-enhancing benefits to boot!

GARDENING THERAPY

Today, topsoil in many areas is devoid of beneficial organisms and contaminated with heavy metals, pesticide accumulation, and other toxins. Such scarcity of one of the planet's most basic compositions can make re-creating the hunter-gatherer experience a little tricky sometimes. If you do not currently have direct access to rich, loamy, nutrient-rich soil, you can easily acquire some at your local gardening supply store. Naturally, my next suggestion is that you dig into that rich, dark soil and start a garden.

If space is an issue for you, consider a square-foot garden. According to the folks over at SquareFootGardening.com, square-foot gardening requires up to 80 percent less space than a traditional garden, eliminates all tilling, wedding, and digging, and can harvest up to five times more produce than a conventional garden. In addition, you get to select what you grow and how you grow it, which means no pesticides or chemicals. Alternatively, you can garden from pots on your balcony, or even hang a cloth shoe organizer against a wall on your patio, and fill the pockets with soil and plant herbs. Or look into starting or joining a community co-op garden.

As any gardening enthusiast will tell you, gardening is much more than just maintaining a yard. It's the sun on your shoulders, the nurturing of seedlings, the thoughtful grooming (and pruning) of a creative vision, the witnessing of a living, growing force. It's a labor of love and, for many, a show of true artistry. Gardening is a deeply sensory experience, and I think it touches something innate in the human spirit. Then there's the dirt itself—the beautiful, misunderstood soil. The sensory pleasure of soft, cool crumbling earth between ungloved fingers, the physical, primordial delight of digging and absorbing oneself in the earth. Clearly, even if your horticultural results are ultimately nothing to write home about, there's gratification to be found in the endeavor.

The fact is, whatever gets us down in the dirt, digging in the midst of all those fine microbes, is work worth doing. My neighbor always tells me gardening is "good for the soul." Although I don't have an ounce of the talent she does, I'd have to agree. Research demonstrates that gardening is also good for the mind and body—in ways we might not expect.

Little surprise, I'd say, that researchers in Taiwan found one of the biggest motivations for gardening among one study's participants was the "escape."[18] I

WORM FARMING

The ultimate "get back to the earth" experience might just be vermiculture—the art and science of raising worms to harvest their, uh, waste. It sounds unsavory, but the results will make you a believer. The manure creates a humus-like soil material rich with the natural minerals and microorganisms to support healthy, nutrient-rich vegetation. Many gardeners call it black gold for its ability to nourish your garden, producing yields high in vitamin C and many minerals like magnesium, phosphorus, and potassium.

Here's the how-to: Choose a bin to support your worm farm. Drill holes in the bottom and sides. Insert wire mesh dense enough to keep the worms in. Start with some good quality organic soil and a collection of red wiggler worms. Keep the soil moist, cool, and shielded from light sources. Feed your farm regularly with table scraps of cut vegetables and fruits, lettuce, produce peels, eggshells, grass, and tea and coffee grounds. (Don't use dairy, meat, onion, or citrus.) Keep the soil's pH balanced (you can purchase a pH meter at most garden stores), and you'll keep your worms happy and productive.

would venture to guess this is a universal motivation. Life begins in the garden, so they say. The rest—worry, conflict, stress—simply dissolves in the landscape.

In a Netherlands-based study, stressed participants were divided into two groups—one which read indoors and one which gardened in their allotment plots. Although both groups demonstrated a drop in cortisol, the gardening participants showed a much steeper drop and fared much better in terms of mood.[19]

Want more? In a Texas A&M survey, gardeners reported more physical activity, claimed more energy, and rated their overall health higher than non-gardeners. Those who described themselves as gardeners showed a higher level of life satisfaction than those who said they didn't garden. Numerous studies demonstrate both physical and mental health benefits for older adults, including higher vegetable intake, better hand strength, and higher self-esteem.[20]

Gardening at times seems antithetical to modern society. It requires time and patience—both scarce commodities these days. Many of us, however, invest just that for the sake of experiencing life in the garden. In a way, we tend to ourselves within the garden's rows and patches. We participate in unpredictable cycles and risks of nature, with its messy interactions and unsure outcomes, the kind of stuff modernity so often edits out, causing us to miss out on much of life's vitality. Gardening, in a sense, helps us reclaim those encounters.

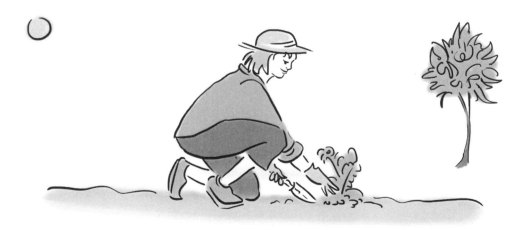

SECTION SUMMARY

The Wild Within. Our primal ancestors lived an earthy, sensual existence on the wide-open African savanna, surrounded by the sights, sounds, smells, and sensations of rain, vegetation, birds, and yes, even the odor of predators. We, on the other hand, encounter pollution and soot, recirculated indoor air, and the high-decibel noises of civilization. Though our connection with the wild is far removed, our genes still expect age-old, nature-based inputs. Amid natural surroundings, our senses heighten, and the abundant stress-relieving negative ions generally found in such settings helps melt away stress and energize mind and body.

Reclaiming the Outdoors. Even the most impacted urban areas have outdoor escapes to satisfy your hardwired need for nature. Visit your local park, zoo, hike or bike trails. At the very least, create an inviting space on your balcony, porch, or yard to eat, play, or lie around in. In addition to reclaiming more outdoor time, bring some of the outdoors into your living space with house plants that act as natural air scrubbers and purifiers. Remember, reconnecting with the wild requires a deep familiarity with the land in which you reside. Get out of the car and explore your neighborhood and community on foot. Invest time, interest, and attention to the discovery of the new to be found within the old and familiar.

Play Dirty. Grok existed in an intimate relationship with the soil, consuming germs and other microbes at every meal. It is in fact how he replanted his gut with beneficial bacteria and kick-started his immune system. This is how our immune system works. The more microbes you encounter (within reason, of course), the more antibodies your body creates, and thus the stronger it becomes, ready to do fast work on harmful bacteria, viruses, fungi, and protozoa that it inevitably comes in contact with. In an overly clean society, however, we end up hampering this process. Increases in allergies, asthma, autism, obesity, type 1 diabetes, mood disorders, multiple sclerosis, inflammatory bowel disease, and other conditions related to systemic inflammation or autoimmune dysfunction are conditions of the industrialized world, partially blamed on our lack of exposure to dirt and bacteria. Ditch antibacterial cleaners, relax your hygiene standards in general, and make a concerted effort to engage with dirt and other organic matter.

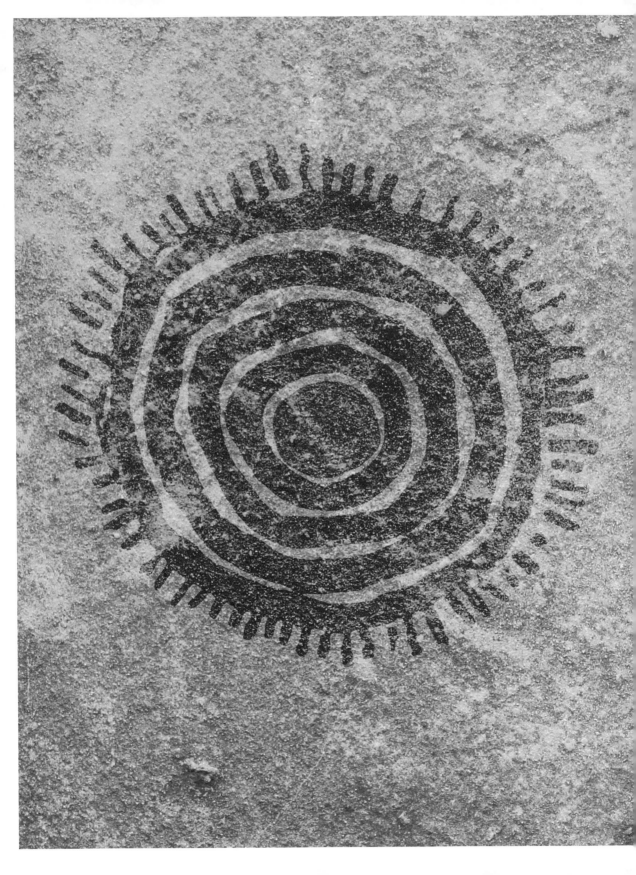

THE DAILY RHYTHM CONNECTION

THE DAILY RHYTHM OF LIFE. Or the daily grind, depending on how disconnected you've become. Long before the arrival of hominids, the genes of every living thing came to rely on the daily cycle of the planet, the rising and setting of the sun. It is a circuit we cannot escape. Among the many intricate hormonal and neurotransmitter interactions we rely on, the production of melatonin comes with nightfall, while serotonin comes with the break of day. Within this ancient order, we've created an artificial microcosm, one made up of glaring lights, computers, digital gadgets, text messages, emails, Tweets, and Facebook updates that rule our days and overstimulate our nights. All these are meant to connect us, but—irony of ironies—they prevent us from forging deeper, more meaningful bonds. This section will show you how to honor your circadian rhythm and use technology without it consuming you. You will learn to slow down, take notice, and breathe deeply. For in the grand scheme of things, the only thing you truly own is this single moment, right here and right now. The connection here is learning what you can do with this moment to positively and naturally affect those that follow.

I've loved the stars too fondly to be fearful of the night.

GALILEO GALILEI

HONORING THE SUN

PERHAPS NO OTHER NATURAL FORCE has a more powerful effect on all living things than the consistent rising and setting of the sun. It is the sun, after all, that rules over our circadian rhythm, our internal, approximately twenty-four-hour cycle of biochemical, physiological, and behavioral processes. Every living thing, from fungus to bacteria to plant to animal, has a circadian rhythm. As you approach your usual bedtime, your body anticipates what's coming, and your bloodstream and brain reach their highest concentration of adenosine, a sleep-promoting neurotransmitter. Simultaneously, your body begins to kick out melatonin and reduce its core temperature, hitting its lowest point in the second half of your normal sleep schedule—around the time when melatonin will, incidentally, be at its highest. Your best sleep, not surprisingly, results from staying on course with your natural circadian rhythm.

For 2.5 million years of human history, and tens of millions of years before that, our genes have grown solidly, and inescapably, accustomed to the light and dark cycles of Earth. When we fail to obtain adequate sleep, we decrease our ability to process even moderate levels of oxidative stress. The impact leads to faster aging and measurable neurological decline. Our circadian rhythm governs our patterns of sleep, hunger, and wakefulness, as well as the flow of numerous hormones that support all aspects of health and wellbeing.

During sleep, elevated levels of testosterone, human growth hormone, and other adaptive hormones pulse through your body, a critical nighttime process that repairs organs and strengthens and rebuilds muscle. What's more, your immune system's white blood cells kick into high gear, with macrophages and leukocytes multiplying rapidly, thus inducing healthy flora to prevail over harmful bacteria. Your brain is also a beneficiary. The various phases of light-to-heavy sleep each night help your brain organize short- and long-term memories and fine-tune other cognitive processes like problem solving. Brain scientists call this *synaptic homeostasis*, but you might consider it a luxury spa makeover for the brain.

Just like a day at the spa refreshes your body, a night of sleep refreshes your synapses, the spaces located between nerve cells that allow the cells to communicate with each other. They respond to myriad, often overwhelming stimulation during your waking hours. The more enriched (or stimulating) your days are, the more your synapses grow, but they can only take so much before they exhaust. At the end of a busy day, when we say we're "fried" or "drained," we're speaking literally. Under ideal conditions, you retire for the evening, and by morning, on cue with the rising of the sun, you awake naturally refreshed and rejuvenated, your synapses returned to their baseline values.

Of course, few of us these days enter our nightly slumber under ideal conditions. Stress, poor diet, sleep medications, cluttered sleeping environments, erratic bedtimes often disturb the delicate hormonal systems that restore the mind and body, to say nothing of excessive artificial light and digital stimulation after dark, when our circadian rhythm should signal us to wind down. Consider also the effects of air travel that unnaturally compresses or extends your days, and alarm clocks that force you awake. This is especially harmful before sunrise because it throws off your hardwired circadian-influenced hormone patterns.

A 2006 Harvard School of Public Health survey found that 75 percent of Americans suffer from some form of sleep difficulty, and a shocking 40 percent are

YOU ARE HARDWIRED *to fall asleep shortly after sunset.*

MODERN DISCONNECT: *excessive light and digital stimulation after dark.*

PRIMAL CONNECTION: *embrace mellow, low-light evenings; create an optimal sleep.*

seriously deficient, receiving less than five hours of sleep per night. By no small coincidence are the sleep deprived either suffering from, or are at increased risk for, numerous health problems, including hypertension, suppressed immune function, sexual dysfunction, thyroid dysfunction, premature aging, cancer, and heart disease. Mental health suffers, too. In addition to exhaustion, sleep deficiency is linked to aggression, depression, irritability, ADHD, and mood disturbance disorders. Even just a single night of deficient sleep can cause your level of cortisol to increase for prolonged periods of time, compromising your ability to handle the stress of a busy day.

Now let's take a look at how the hormones and neurotransmitters that influence your circadian rhythm are supposed to work. Soon after it gets dark, melatonin levels rise—a hardwired process known as *dim light melatonin onset* (DLMO). When you feel drowsy, that's your melatonin working its magic on you. Its job is to mellow you out by relaxing your brain waves and muscles while simultaneously lowering your body temperature, blood pressure, heart rate, and breathing rate. It's also a powerful antioxidant, so it's doing a fair share of cleaning house, too. Come morning, the rising sun triggers the suppression of this powerful hormone and increases the production of serotonin, a neurotransmitter that helps boost mood and energy levels during your waking hours. This, ladies and gentlemen, is your circadian rhythm at its best.

BASK IN THE WARM GLOW

For most of human history, nighttime meant darkness. I'm talking about real, permeating darkness. Camping darkness. Small-country-road-with-the-car-lights-out darkness. For our ancestors as recently as a couple hundred years ago, this kind of nighttime darkness lasted up to fourteen hours (well, it does today, too, but we mask it with lighting). Artificial lighting back then meant candles and firewood.

Today, in addition to artificial lighting, we possess computers, televisions, and digital gadgets that emit *blue light*, named for the sustained and vivid hue on the electromagnetic spectrum, which runs from infrared to ultraviolet. The bluer the light, the more intense it registers on the Kelvin temperature scale. For reference, candle light, which falls in the red-orange-yellow area of the spectrum, burns at 1800K; incandescent indoor light registers around 3000K; ultraviolet noon sunlight comes in at 5500K; and the light emitted from most computer monitors registers a whopping 6500K!

Apologies to Thomas Edison, Steve Jobs, Bill Gates, and the rest, but they did play a role in thrusting us violently—genetically speaking—into the Digital Age. Exposure to artificial light after dark suppresses melatonin's DLMO effect and triggers instead an elevation of cortisol and other stress hormones. So, why should this concern you? Because this unnatural spike in cortisol not only keeps you from falling asleep, but also causes sugar cravings, elevates ghrelin secretion (which stimulates hunger), elevates insulin levels (which promotes fat storage while you sleep), and compromises the effects of leptin, an important hormone that regulates appetite and fat metabolism hormone. Translation: Blast your retinas with artificial light, and you'll get the late-night munchies. And you'll signal your genes to store these calories as body fat.

The synergy of light, appetite, and fat storage is actually a desirable evolutionary process kicking in. Our ancestors stayed up later in the summers eating carbs in the form of seasonal fruits, vegetables, and tubers. This triggered hormonal processes that prompted their bodies to start storing fat, a desired effect when considering the long, cold, dark winters that lay ahead. Bear in mind, these were times when winter meant zero carb availability, meaning, instead of burning stored glycogen and muscle in the winter, our ancestors burned mostly fat. Most people today, however, are locked into a fat storage pattern year-round, thanks to a high-sugar, grain-based diet and artificially lengthened "days."

Over a lifetime, excessive exposure to blue light can result in a variety of degenerative eye diseases, including cataracts and macular degeneration. Furthermore, researchers believe that a lifetime of excessive light exposure (and the related suppression of melatonin) is harmful not just to your eyes and sleep cycles, but can also increase the risk of many forms of cancer.

To that end, your best bet is to make a sincere effort to get by with the absolute minimum amount of artificial light possible when indoors—even during the day. This will help ease eye fatigue and potential long-term damage from excessive blue-light exposure. Don't be afraid of actual sunlight, however. Just as it did for Grok, sunlight ignites serotonin production and delivers vitamin D, which, as we'll discuss shortly, plays a critical role in healthy metabolic, cardiac, immune, skeletal, and neurological function.

OVERCOMING JET LAG

In the evolution of our genetic blueprint, it was never remotely contemplated that we would travel far enough to disrupt our circadian rhythms. Little wonder, then, that changing three, four, or nine time zones in as little as half a day can wreak havoc on all your delicate internal "wiring" and hormonal systems, leaving you exhausted and with a weakened immune system. If you're a frequent flyer, it can even increase your risk for cancer, ulcers, and sleep disorders. Now, this isn't reason to stop traveling; just be aware of the risks and take some smart precautions:

Set your watch to your new time zone as soon as you board the plane. When traveling east, look for flights that leave late in the day. Treat the flight as a short night and a short day. Treat long flights going west as a very long day (or a very long night, depending on when you leave).

Avoid sleeping pills on the plane. They will not provide quality sleep and can interfere with your adjustment upon arrival. Instead, use a neck pillow to cradle your head; drink lots of water and avoid alcohol; and get up, walk, and stretch occasionally.

Put in an aerobic workout as soon a you reach your destination. Avoid the temptation to drink a glass of wine or take a nap; instead, spend thirty minutes getting into a comfortable aerobic zone of 55–75 percent of maximum heart rate. Don't exceed 75 percent or you will stimulate cortisol production, which is already elevated from the stress of the flight.

Drink at least four glasses of water on the first day of arrival. This will help counter the pronounced dehydrating effect of flying.

Go to bed at the same time as everyone else in your new time zone. Take 3 to 6 milligrams of melatonin an hour before you plan to fall asleep to make that possible. If you need to, take it each of the next two nights as well. By the third night, you should be acclimated.

So, as the sun begins to set, that's your cue to minimize your light exposure, especially blue light. Hey, it isn't that bad. Low-temperature light—such as that found in fire flame—has no effect on melatonin production and facilitates relaxation of the central nervous system even more than lowering general ambient light. This makes romantic candlelit evenings a great way to stay aligned with your circadian rhythm. Grok really knew what he was doing when he built his campfires!

For those nights when it simply isn't practical to live by the light of fire, consider purchasing yellow-, orange-, or red-tinted light bulbs (often marketed as "bug bulbs" at home supply stores), and switch out lamps in your home as you see fit to afford low-light evenings. Another effective strategy, particularly if you are working or watching computer and television screens after dark, is to wear yellow- or orange-tinted glasses with UV protection. Light-colored lenses let sufficient light in so you can see fine, but, with the familiar UV designation (indicating protection from the sun's ultraviolet rays), they protect you from the damaging effects that indoor blue light has on your melatonin release. You can purchase a quality pair of yellow- or orange-tinted sport lenses from leading sunglass manufacturers such as Smith Sport USA, or acquire inexpensive safety glasses of similar colors from a big-box home-supply store or Internet resources.

SWEET DREAMS ARE MADE OF THESE

Your bedroom should be considered a sanctuary devoted to sleep, relaxation, and intimacy. TVs, computers, clutter, including stacks of mail, piles of laundry, and old magazines, have no place here. Even your smart phone is off limits, unless perhaps you're using an app to play soothing nature sounds. Add plenty of plants to purify the air. Maybe even a few candles—that's a nice touch, too. You want your sleeping environment to be warm and inviting; however, when it comes to the actual temperature, you definitely want to lean toward the cool side. Evolution has programmed us to sleep in environments that are cooler by night than they are by day. Bundle up under the covers, but keep your head in cooler-than-daylight temperatures. Research suggests that the optimal room temperature for sleeping lies somewhere between 60 and 68 degrees Fahrenheit (16 to 20 Celsius), so set your thermostat accordingly. Or go truly Primal by cracking open a window and letting the fresh, cool air drift you off to sleep.

As for bedding, our ancestors likely made the best of soft sand, piles of leaves, or even just the bare ground. While some Primal enthusiasts tout the benefits of firm sleeping surfaces, personal preference should guide you to the most comfortable bedding and pillow setup. Spend some time experimenting with different options and splurge for the best—after all, you (hopefully) spend a third of your life in bed! Since back and neck pain are so common these days, it's important to observe correct sleeping positions, as detailed in the sidebar for the Gokhale Method for Lying Down (see page 146).

When it's time for lights out, your sleeping environment should be completely dark. Do whatever it takes here. Install blackout curtains or room-darkening blinds. If light streams in through cracks of your windows, cover them with heavy dark fabric or paper. Shield LCD readouts, wedge a towel under the door to block interference from other rooms, and keep a flashlight handy instead of plugged-in nightlights. Use a sleep mask when you sleep or nap during times when it's not dark outside, or when you can't completely darken the room for whatever reason. Yes, this is a huge deal, even if you claim to be an easygoing sleeper.

Research has shown that it's not just your eyes that are light sensitive, but the entire surface of your skin as well. Even a single beam of light hitting the back of your knee has been demonstrated to disrupt melatonin levels and upset your circadian rhythm. Consequently, once your body fully acclimates to sleeping and waking with the cycle of the sun, even the most aggressive blackout effort probably won't stop you from gracefully waking at the break of dawn. For one, lighter sleeping cycles predominate in the morning. And secondly, environmental cues called *zeitgebers*—German for "time giver"—typically stir you out of sleep. These cues also help sync your circadian rhythm, and in addition to daylight, include warming temperatures and the sounds of nature such as chirping birds.

THE HOURS OF THE NIGHT

Although it might feel like it some days, hitting the pillow doesn't mean an instantaneous plunge into cataleptic nothingness. Sleep follows a progressive spectrum of sorts. We likely all recall the REM (Rapid Eye Movement) and non-REM designations from our middle school health classes. The picture is a bit more complicated than that, but those categories represent the bones of it.

Essentially, the body moves through three stages of non-REM sleep called N1, N2, and N3, proceeding eventually to REM sleep, characterized by dreaming. The typical pattern we follow is N1, N2, N3, N2, and then REM. A complete cycle through this pattern lasts about ninety minutes, and the cycle repeats several times throughout the night. Early in the evening, your N3 deep-sleep cycles are prolonged, and your N1 and REM sleep cycles are relatively short. As you progress toward awakening in the morning, your deep sleep cycles are shorter and your lighter sleep cycles lengthen—making it easier to awaken refreshed and energized after a complete cycling through all the necessary phases or restoration.

Phase N1 represents the initial switch in brain-wave frequency. It's the stage in which you feel like you're mostly under but can still sense the presence of the exterior world. It characterizes most surreptitious office naps that people think no one will notice—until your head slips off the hand that was holding it up. It's the stage in which you scare yourself (and your sleeping partner) with those annoying sudden jerks. From there, N2 takes you down enough that any residual awareness of your environment is gone. We spend about 50 percent of our sleep in this stage throughout the night. During this stage, we consolidate the learning of complex motor skills and upload information processed during REM sleep into long-term memory. Those hours of piano practice or shooting three-pointers get hardwired into your nervous system circuitry. The process, known as long-term potentiation (LTP), becomes, as the complexity of the learning increases, more dependent on good sleep. So, when NBA players and concert saxophonists take their customary naps before evening performances, they are getting a potentiation boost for the complex motor skills they must master.

Finally, at N3 you reach deep, slow-wave sleep. This is where we spend about 30 percent of our total sleep time. Adaptive hormones flow at peak levels, and macronutrients are synthesized efficiently so that your bones, muscles, and organs are repaired and replenished. Slowed brain function at this stage helps clear your mind of unnecessary clutter and insignificant memories. Since slow-wave sleep predominates early in your sleeping period, it's critical to get to bed on

YOU ARE HARDWIRED *to awake naturally refreshed.*

MODERN DISCONNECT: *alarm clocks that awake you in a state of fight or flight.*

PRIMAL CONNECTION: *wakening with the rising sun, thanks to mellow evenings and Primal sleeping habits.*

GOKHALE METHOD FOR LYING DOWN

Lower your sacrum to your sleeping surface, lay your palms on the ground, and slowly lower yourself back, taking care to lengthen your spine actively—vertebra by vertebra—by pushing through your hands and unrolling and elongating your spine. Take care not to tuck your pelvis. With your head and shoulders on the pillow, gently elongate your neck, and relax and lower your shoulders. If sleeping on your back is difficult, turn on your side. Just make sure that you don't sway or excessively arch the back when lengthening the spine. And avoid curling into a fetal position, as you will compress your spine and stress the spinal discs.

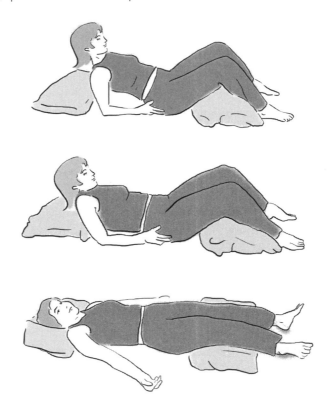

time. As an old sleep proverb states, "An hour before midnight is worth two after." Keep that in mind next time you're tempted to stay up for just a few more emails or a late-night talk show.

We spend about 20 percent of our sleeping hours in REM. In this state, your muscles are paralyzed to keep you from acting out your dreams while your racing mind consolidates and processes information from your day for storage into

> **REM sleep helps to improve spatial, perceptual, and visual skills.**

long-term memory. REM sleep helps to improve spatial, perceptual, and visual skills, as well as sort out emotional experiences and stressful events, improve neural connections that strengthen memory, and replenish important mood and cognitive-boosting neurotransmitters like serotonin and dopamine.

While it's nice to achieve the tidy, repeating pattern of N cycles into REM cycles, don't be alarmed should you spin out of a sleep cycle sometime during the night. Researchers believe that our primal ancestors likely engaged in biphasic or possibly even polyphasic sleeping habits instead of sleeping in one uninterrupted stretch as most of us do (or try to do) today. Their night's sleep was likely interrupted to tend to the fire, feed and care for infants, or keep watch for danger.

According to historian A. Roger Ekirch, the author of *At Day's Close: Night in Times Past*, segmented sleep predominated up until the Industrial Revolution. Ekirch's groundbreaking research, validated by more than five hundred references in historical documents, suggests that we have a natural preference for polyphasic sleep and that many modern sleep problems stem from overriding this preference with too much artificial light after dark. As a result, we retire for the evening much later than we would otherwise, and try to make up the time by sleeping in one interrupted stretch throughout the night.

According to Ekirch, after catching a few hours of quality shut-eye, people before the Industrial Age would naturally stir out of sleep in the middle of the night and engage in assorted activities such as sex, prayer, writing, interpreting dreams, visiting neighbors, and smoking tobacco. The unscrupulous engaged in petty crime, but most generally enjoyed the nocturnal free time that was, for the working class, virtually nonexistent during the day. This wakeful segment lasted one to two hours, followed by another good chunk of sleep lasting till sunrise.

Ekirch and other sleep scientists believe there are numerous health benefits from segmented sleep. Studies show increased levels of the hormone prolactin during periods of late-night wakefulness. While commonly associated with lactation, prolactin provides hundreds of other benefits, including regulating immune and endocrine functions, and promoting gratification and relaxation after sex (countering the arousing effects of dopamine that occur before sex).

The idea that we are programmed for biphasic or polyphasic sleep is not a new one. In 1992, the National Institute of Mental Health conducted an experiment that involved depriving a group of sleep subjects of light for weeks at a time, causing the subjects to fall into a segmented sleep routine very similar to that described in Ekirch's historical diaries, court documents, medical books, and literature.

Segmented sleep should not be confused with the common condition of *sleep maintenance insomnia*, which occurs when people awaken in the middle of the night and have difficulty falling back asleep. In fact, findings suggest waking up regularly in the night might not constitute the sleep disorder it's commonly made out to be. In other words, it may be natural—and not all bad. Just don't turn on any blue lights that could suppress your evening melatonin.

If you have to get up and move around, replace your plug-in nightlights with a small flashlight at your bedside, and, if your want to be ultra diligent, tape it with some red cellophane over the lens to stay within the warm-light range. Or wear yellow-orange lenses and use a low-light, lightweight headlamp, essentially a strap-on "miner's light," or use a specially designed book light. Yes, I admit the miner's light is quirky. But it works, and it's great for mellowing out the kids at bedtime. You can pick up an inexpensive one from a hardware store or check out one of the fancy models from the Petzl brand. But do whatever it takes to get cozy and minimize light as much as possible during these mid-night awakenings. And as soon as you feel drowsy, just shut things down and return to sleep.

Regarding the optimal amount of sleep you should get, genetics as well as your levels of activity, stress, fatigue, and general mental and physical health all influence what your magic number is. While conventional wisdom's eight-hour recommendation is reasonable and safe, an often overlooked element of optimal sleep is the need to vary your sleeping habits in accordance with the seasonal sunlight exposure at your latitude.

In the book *Lights Out: Sleep, Sugar, and Survival*, authors T.S. Wiley and Bent Formby make a strong case for getting 9.5 hours per night for six to seven months of the year, and eight or less during the longer days of summer. Those living in the tropics require less variation, while those living near the polar regions need more variation between summer and winter sleep patterns.

Granted, 9.5 hours might seem excessive considering the hectic twenty-four-hour cycles we push through today. But consider this: when you honor this connection, you are more productive and focused during the peak hours of the day. You get more done faster, easier, better, more creatively. Set a Primal Connection priority of winding things down after dark with just a bare minimum of lighting and little, if any, digital stimulation. Enjoy quiet, calming activities instead such as neighborhood strolls, conversation, reading, or board games with the family. Mellow, low-light evenings should adequately induce the effects of DLMO to get you settled into sleep soon after dark. For those in the continental USA or living at similar latitudes, a good time to go to sleep is somewhere within one to two hours of sunset during the summer months and within four to five hours during the winter months.

GOOD MORNING, SUNSHINE!

As we have just learned, your body's biological clock, better known in the scientific community as the *suprachiasmatic nucleus* (SCN), gently tucks you in to sleep at night with melatonin, and awakens you refreshed the next morning with serotonin. If you are strongly aligned with your circadian rhythm, your morning hormonal process works by first receiving light through your retina. From there, a signal travels along the optic nerve to your SCN and swiftly sends signals to other regions of your brain, including the pineal gland, which activates the release of serotonin. This high-energy neurotransmitter makes you feel alert and happy, and helps you learn and process memory. Not enough of it and you suffer, namely from depression. Levels of the stress hormone cortisol begin to increase within the first thirty minutes of your awakening as well. While cortisol is often maligned as health-compromising when produced in excess, this morning bump is a desirable genetic mechanism that prepares you for the energy demands of a busy day. In fact, the serotonin-cortisol effect is most pronounced when you awake close to sunrise, so early risers have an added advantage.

If waking up naturally on schedule in the morning is difficult for you, try moving your bed near a window that receives sunlight. This is a good option if you can keep your room decently dark during the night. If the environmental cues of chirping birds, trickling water, or ocean waves are a lacking feature near your home, research suggests that nature sounds produced by a variety of sophisticated alarm clocks and cell phone apps might help. Some models emit a gradually increasing glow a half an hour or so before your scheduled wake-up time, and others provide your choice of soft ambient sound. Guaranteed, you'll awake more gracefully using this hack than by the artificial and disruptive noise of a traditional alarm. Such rude awakenings stimulate an undesirable spike of stress hormones, in contrast to the optimal elevation caused by sunlight. You want to wake refreshed, not in a state of fight or flight.

SLEEP AND WAKE HACKS

Sometimes you need to manipulate the cycle of your circadian rhythm to your benefit, particularly if you are among the many folks—shift workers, parents caring for infants, and so on—who routinely require sleep during daylight hours.

Sleep masks. Also known as blindfolds, this sleeping solution creates a dark environment anytime you want to induce or prolong sleep. Check with your local drug store or DreamEssentials.com.

Noise-canceling machines. Fans, air purifiers, digital nature sounds from your music device, or noise-canceling machines counter potentially disruptive, narrow-frequency external noise such as barking dogs, a snoring partner, and loud voices that can interfere with sleep.

Power naps. A natural, circadian-influenced energy lull happens about seven to eight hours after you wake. Assuming you wake near sunrise, by early afternoon you may on certain days experience a dip in energy. During this lull, your body temperature drops to its lowest point during daylight hours, making early afternoon an ideal naptime. Don't be dissuaded by the common sentiment that napping will throw off your evening sleep. No research supports this, and in fact some research suggests otherwise, that a well-timed twenty-minute catnap (or even a big-time nap of up to ninety minutes) can actually improve your evening sleep, even if you suffer from insomnia.

Light therapy boxes. We've talked about minimizing light, but if you live in a sun-challenged environment, have a work schedule that is at odds with the sun, or suffer from seasonal mood disorders, consider a light therapy box that mimics ultraviolet daylight and can help you regulate your circadian rhythm. Brief exposure to a light box when you wake can stimulate the production of serotonin and other awakening hormones. Purchase a high-quality unit with a certifiable output level of around 10,000 lux and an effective UV filter to ensure safety.

Tanning beds. Another way to work around seasonal mood disorders. Be careful not to go overboard and chase the high with this hack. Consider brief exposure only, about twenty minutes a week. Make absolutely sure you patronize a facility that uses the latest technology; that is, low- or medium-pressure lamps that emit a balance of UVA and UVB radiation similar to sunlight. Ask your salon about these sorts of lamps. If they don't know what you're taking about, choose another salon! I strongly recommend covering your face with a towel while you fake bake, since our faces get plenty of sun exposure and are most susceptible to wrinkling and carcinoma over a lifetime. At the very least, protect your lips and wear goggles over your eyes.

F.lux. If you must work on your computer after sunset, take regular screen breaks to rest your eyes and brain. And don't forget to use your yellow-tinted sunglasses to cut down the blue-light exposure! Downloading F.lux (Stereopsis.com), a free computer program that works by warming the color temperature of your computer display to a more mellow pink-colored hue after the sun sets in your area, is another great option for late-night writing jags.

VITAMIN D AND THE SUNNY SIDE OF LIFE

No discussion of the rising and setting of the sun would be complete without acknowledging the powerful impact direct sunlight has on the production of vitamin D, which, as previously stated, is technically not a vitamin but another potent and essential hormone. Within your epidermis, enzymatic "biofactories" convert cholesterol derivatives to vitamin D when UVB rays of sunlight hit your bare skin. (Yes, cholesterol! Like sunlight, our bodies would not be able to function without it.) The newly created vitamin D is then distributed to receptors located within cells throughout your body, playing a central role in metabolizing calcium; strengthening immunity, cardiac, and neurological function; and, ultimately, gene expression.

Overall, some two thousand genes are influenced—or turned on—by vitamin D, triggering elevated levels of beta-endorphins and serotonin. We're talking about some serious feel-good stuff here! Vitamin D also works to regulate cell growth and renewal, particularly by acting on the P53 gene, the appropriately named "DNA proofreader" gene, which is responsible for overseeing hundreds of millions of daily cell replications. It's also involved in apoptosis, the natural self-destruction of superfluous or damaged cells before they become malignant. In the absence of vitamin D, however, the P53 gene will down-regulate—or turn off—and the risk of many forms of cancer, including melanoma, will dramatically increase.

Without question, the sun has left a deep imprint on our genetic makeup and primary biological processes, dating back some 350 million years, when vertebrates first left the calcium-rich sea for land. Vitamin D synthesis set the stage for creatures to proliferate and become more complex with healthy, mineralized skeletons. Evolutionary biologists report that vitamin D's ability to boost immune function and destroy invading organisms has been conserved in the genome of all primates for over 60 million years.

So, it's pretty darn clear that receiving adequate vitamin D is an essential component of being a healthy, happy *Homo sap sap*. And yet a 2009 study published in the *Archives of Internal Medicine* reveals that 77 percent of Americans have insufficient levels of it in their bodies. In fact, we're learning that vitamin D deficiency is one of the most disastrous disconnects in modern society. How did this happen? How is it that in the beginning of the twenty-

> **Vitamin D's ability to boost immune function and destroy invading organisms has been conserved in the genome of all primates for over 60 million years.**

first century, in developed countries, we are seeing a resurgence of all sorts of debilitating health problems, including a rise in cancer and a return of rickets?

Our sedentary indoor lifestyle is one big reason. And when we *do* go outdoors, flawed conventional wisdom encourages us to shun the sun, and cover up and slather sunscreen all over our bods, from head to toe. We're warned of wrinkles and skin cancers with ominous names like malignant melanoma and basal cell carcinoma. But the reality is no scientific evidence links regular, *moderate* sun exposure to any form of skin cancer. Only *excessive* sun exposure presents a skin cancer risk, and even then mainly for carcinoma—the easily treatable condition—and not melanoma, the far more serious condition.

For every skin cancer diagnosis attributed to excessive sun exposure, there are fifty-five more cancer diagnoses attributed to insufficient sunlight. University of California researchers believe that more than sixty thousand annual cases of colon and breast cancer worldwide can be prevented simply by increasing the intake of vitamin D.[1] In fact, recent studies link vitamin D deficiency as the root cause of other health complaints such as depression, fibromyalgia, and muscle and joint pain. Think about that the next time you layer on a thick glob of sunscreen. One with a Sun Protection Factor (SPF) of 8 compromises vitamin D by 90 percent, while SPF 30 blocks 99 percent of vitamin D. (Never mind that a good Primal Blueprint diet and, guess what, adequate vitamin D, bolsters our natural sunburn and sun damage defenses.)

Obviously, sun exposure is all about striking the right balance. Too little or too much, and you pay the consequences. So, how much is enough? And what's the sensible approach?

YOU ARE HARDWIRED *for your body to manufacture vitamin D by way of sun exposure.*

MODERN DISCONNECT: *an indoor-dominant lifestyle and paranoia about the sun.*

PRIMAL CONNECTION: *sufficient sun exposure over large skin surface areas, or supplement as needed.*

The darker the natural coloring of your skin, hair, and eyes, the more melanin pigment you possess. Melanin is a natural chemical in your body that protects your skin from excess solar radiation (UVA ultraviolet light), so the more you have, the more you can enjoy risk-free sun time. Those with red hair and extremely fair skin have difficultly manufacturing melanin. If you have fair-to-medium skin pigment, you can easily synthesize vitamin D, but you burn easily. Strive for a slight in-season tan—somewhere between ten to twenty minutes of direct sunlight daily over 25 to 50 percent of your body. Avoid burning, and you will be safe. But even at the equator, the early morning and late afternoon sun is not intense enough to support vitamin D production, so your window of opportunity typically lies between 10 a.m. to 3 p.m. only during the periods of mid-spring to mid-autumn in the latitudes where most North Americans and Europeans live. A good in-season strategy, represented by that slight tan, should keep enough vitamin D cycling through your system year-round. This is because your fat cells store enough vitamin D to get you through the winter months.

The darker your eyes and skin, the more time you need to spend in the sun to manufacture optimal amounts of vitamin D. This has become a serious complication for those of African descent living indoor-dominant lifestyles outside the tropics. Recent findings show that African American males have an 89 percent greater risk of cancer mortality than white men, and have particularly high rates of digestive tract cancers (colon, rectum, mouth, esophagus, stomach, and pancreas) that are strongly linked to vitamin D deficiency.

DIALING IN YOUR VITAMIN D STRATEGY

Manufacturing vitamin D from sunlight occurs only when ultraviolet radiation is greater than 3 on the UV index, something that is affected by numerous variables: high altitudes (the more intense the UV, the more vitamin D production), reflectiveness of ground surface (light reflected off sand, snow, concrete and water increases vitamin D production; the opposite for grass and other less reflective surfaces), pollution (minimizes UV, and therefore lessens vitamin D production) and obviously time of day, time of year, and your skin pigment. Since "maintain a slight tan" might be too vague of a recommendation for something this critical to your health, it's helpful to have a basic understanding of how to optimize your vitamin D production, predominantly through sun exposure.

Dr. Michael Holick, author of *The Vitamin D Solution* and one of the world's leading authorities on vitamin D health, recommends a maximum safe sun exposure time of *half the amount of time it takes to sustain a slight (pink) sunburn that is noticeable twenty-four hours later.* This benchmark—which Dr. Holick refers to as one minimal erythemal dose (1 MED) automatically factors in all the aforementioned variables. For example, a redhead on a white-sand beach in Southern California in mid-summer can burn his or her skin in a matter of minutes. Someone of medium skin pigment playing on a grass field in New York City in the fall, however, can spend a couple hours in the direct sunlight without burning.

If you obtain sun exposure equivalent to half of 1 MED (half of burn time) over approximately half of your skin surface, your body will produce an estimated 2,000 to 4,000 International Units (I.U.) of sun-obtained vitamin D, which, incidentally, lasts twice as long in your body as a vitamin D supplement of the same amount. Knowing this, it becomes clear how insignificant dietary vitamin D sources are, and how important it is to expose large skin surface areas of your body to sunlight frequently during the months of peak solar intensity at your latitude. Naturally, your half a MED exposure time will be an estimate, since there is no reason to sustain a burn in order to pinpoint your 1 MED time!

By the way, if you are imagining your dermatologist cringing at the suggestion to expose your fair skin to more rays, go ahead and cover sunscreen on your face, neck, and hands whenever you spend time in the sun. Protecting these vulnerable areas from potential wrinkling and cancerous growths will not materially hamper your body from manufacturing vitamin D. This is because your face and hands represent only a small fraction of your total skin surface and total vitamin D manufacturing potential. Focus on your legs (36 percent of total skin surface), back (18 percent), abdomen and chest (18 percent), and arms (18 percent) for vitamin D production, since they have far less risk of chronic exposure damage and loads of potential for vitamin D production.

YOU ARE HARDWIRED *with skin pigment aligned with the latitude of your ancestral homeland.*

MODERN DISCONNECT: *living farther from the equator than your ancestors.*

PRIMAL CONNECTION: *more sun exposure and possible supplementation, especially in winter.*

Still, for a variety of reasons, many of us find it a challenge to expose large areas of our bodies to the sun at midday. For example, you may live at a latitude that is incongruent with our skin pigment and ancestral heritage. Or you may find the sun's rays in your area are only intense enough to make vitamin D for a portion of the year. In such cases, supplementing with vitamin D can

> ❝ Conventional wisdom has long touted a good old glass of milk for a vitamin D boost, yet it delivers a mere 100 I.U. ❞

be extremely useful to ensure that you maintain healthy blood levels of the nutrient year-round. A typical small capsule might dispense 2,000 I.U. And, since vitamin D can be easily stored in your skin, you can take several pills at a time and not have to worry about regimented daily pill popping. In the winter months when UV intensity is low, I recommend getting an average of 2,000 I.U. of vitamin D per day.

Dr. Holick and other vitamin D advocates recommend that you obtain far more than the paltry US RDA of 200 I.U. per day. Dr. Holick suggests getting 25 to 50 percent of 1 MED over 25 to 50 percent of the skin, two to three times per week. I personally take more because I also love the peripheral feel-good benefits of spending time in the sun. There is zero risk of overdosing on solar vitamin D; your melanin/tanning mechanisms ensure that any potential excess vitamin D is destroyed on the surface of your skin before it enters the bloodstream. Historically, the only real risk of vitamin D toxicity has come from ingesting dangerously high levels of overfortified and mislabeled processed foods.

If you have even a slight suspicion that your lifestyle circumstances put you at risk of vitamin D deficiency, it will be valuable to take a clinical approach to the issue. If you have an office job or commute that prevents you from receiving midday sun, live at a latitude in discord from your ancestors, are obese, a growing youth, or pregnant or lactating, or follow a grain-based diet (which can hinder calcium absorption and thus increase vitamin D requirements), this means you!

First, I highly recommend getting your blood levels tested. Make sure to request the most relevant and accurate test, which is for the circulating form of vitamin D known as 25-hydroxyvitamin D. The test may be called "25-vitamin

D" or "serum 25(OH)D." The best time to get this test is early fall, when your vitamin D levels should be at their highest after a summer of adequate sun exposure. You can order a simple, painless home test from ZRT Laboratory for $75 (ZRTlab.com). Your vitamin D levels are represented in nanograms per milliliter (ng/ml). Dr. Holick categorizes values as follows: Under 20 ng/ml is considered deficient. Under 30 ng/ml is insufficient. The ideal range is 40–60 ng/ml, with anything under 100 ng/ml being acceptable. A level over 150 ng/ml is considered toxic, and virtually impossible to get through sun exposure and sensible eating, as mentioned previously. Second, spend some time calculating your vitamin D manufacturing particulars at this web site:

http://nadir.nilu.no/~olaeng/fastrt/VitD-ez_quartMED.html.

This handy tool allows you to input your variables to calculate a reliable estimate of your vitamin D potential for your particular skin pigment, latitude, time of year, and time of day.

When getting regular and adequate amounts of UV 3 intensity rays over large areas of your skin proves to be a difficult task, diet and supplementation comes into play. You may have heard certain foods touted as vitamin D powerhouses: wild salmon, mackerel, herring, catfish, cod liver oil, eggs. These all provide good nutrition, but they only deliver somewhere between 200 to 1,000 I.U. on a typical serving—not nearly enough to make a dent in the bigger picture of overall vitamin D requirements. Conventional wisdom has long touted a good old glass of milk for a vitamin D boost, yet it delivers a mere 100 I.U. By contrast, when I play one of my summertime, two-hour Ultimate Frisbee matches (playing for the "skins" team, naturally!) at 34 degrees latitude in Los Angeles, with my Scandinavian skin pigment, my body manufactures about 15,000 I.U. of solar vitamin D. Got Milk? No, but thanks anyway!

*If I have ever made any valuable discoveries, it has
been owing more to patient attention, than any other talent.*

ISAAC NEWTON

FINDING FOCUS

WE ARE HARDWIRED TO SOLVE problems. We aren't, however, hardwired to solve problems amid distractions. But for many of us, perpetual distraction is the essence of our existence. We wake up and immediately power up to overflowing email inboxes, instant messages, Tweets, Facebook updates, uploads, and downloads. We then give our attention over to voicemails and text messages, maybe texting while standing in line at the coffee house, walking down the street, or worse, while dining out, completely tuning out other sensory details around us. At home, the average American spends about twenty-eight hours a week zoning out in front of his television set. Funny, our sophisticated technology is meant to help us solve problems, but it seems to have created many more. Eye contact with your computer screen or cell phone might have its advantages, but at the expense of eye contact from real life people around you? Our digital technology is meant to make us better, faster, and more productive, yet it has, for many of us, made us poorer in the process, separating us from the downtime that has been a sacred element of our existence throughout human history.

According to researchers at University of California, San Diego, the average American is exposed to about thirty-four gigabytes—over one hundred thousand words—of daily information.[2] That's like absorbing Tolstoy's *War and Peace* in less than five days. Not that we actually *read* all this information—it hits us from various directions, all vying for our attention in different forms: billboards, junk mail, television, computer, text messaging, and so on. In comparison, we encounter three times the amount of information today as we did in 1960![3] Think about that for a minute. It wasn't that long ago that we were licking stamps and envelopes, tethered to corded phone lines, or using a dial-up Internet connection. No doubt, modern technology offers some pretty awesome conveniences. That said, it's worth looking at how you use it.

Look at how your children use technology as well. According to a widely cited report by the University of Michigan, the average American child today plays outdoors only *four minutes* a day![4] Compare that to an average of 6.5 hours of screen time daily,[5] almost all of which is allocated at the expense of outdoor play that was, until recently, the essence of childhood. Not such a great trade-off when you consider that the American Academy of Pediatrics advocates outdoor play not just to control obesity, but also to advance physical strength and dexterity as well as imagination and cognitive development.

Furthermore, a lack of outdoor activity, says Richard Louv, author of *Last Child in the Woods*, can compromise a child's value of place, ability to feel awe and wonder, and sense of appreciation and stewardship. While it appears there is no going back to simpler times, there is good news: to my knowledge, every form of digital technology in existence has an off switch! And there are still plenty of trees to climb, trails to hike, and bikes to pedal.

Look, I'm a guy who serves up a blog post every single day, so I don't want you to misunderstand this message as a wholesale condemnation of technology. I'm all in favor of technological progress. Advancing ideas and making life easier has been a defining component of human life since Day One. The Digital Age is an era of great progress, empowerment, and unlimited potential. It's mind-blowingly wonderful to look up any topic and have an answer, an image, or a video about it within seconds.

But here's the catch: the more you consume digital technology, the more it consumes you. You're clicking

YOU ARE HARDWIRED *to be keenly aware of your surroundings.*

MODERN DISCONNECT: *overwhelmed with distractions.*

PRIMAL CONNECTION: *power down, unplug, and be present in the moment.*

HOW DO YOU EAT A WOOLLY MAMMOTH?

A beast of a project is staring you in the face, and there you are, struggling to focus—or blowing off the work entirely. You mean well. You have every intention of getting it done. You even know stress and panic await as you put it off until the last minute. This knowledge, however, doesn't motivate you, although you know it should. What's behind this behavior we call procrastination? Why do so many responsible, competent adults of our species chronically set themselves up for the torment of flustered haste when they have adequate time to complete a task with sanity fully intact?

Some blame perfectionism. Others claim they need the last-minute pressure to get motivated. Among the most compelling theories on procrastination is old-fashioned impulsiveness. It makes sense. We're navigating a modern world with brains wired for a hunter-gatherer lifestyle of immediacy. Daily living for our ancestors revolved around pressing needs: hunting and gathering each day to eat, collecting water to drink, building a fire to keep warm. Fast-forward, and we find ourselves dropped into an alien world of long-term projections, goals, schedules, and contracts that don't always offer tangible rewards upon completion.

How, then, do we manipulate our primal minds into getting on the stick? Without the harsh consequences of immediate needs, how do we motivate ourselves? First off, break up a project into steps any caveperson could manage. After all, how do you eat a woolly mammoth? One bite at a time. Then give yourself tangible rewards for getting a particular stage done or a material penalty for not completing it on time. How about giving your friend $100 to hold onto until you make a certain deadline? Give—or withhold from—the primal brain what it wants. It's all about working with your wiring.

(mouse), but things aren't really clicking (brain). Turns out that the more choices you encounter over the course of a day, especially trivial choices, the more stressed you become.

True, lack of discipline is certainly a factor. But there is also an evolutionary impetus behind our tendency toward distractibility: we are hardwired to be drawn to novel details in our environment, particularly in the primitive areas of the brain that process the basics, such as sight and sound. Whenever you encounter a new stimulus, natural opioids trigger the brain's reward system by flooding it with a release of dopamine, giving you an immediate rush and

> **We joke about the 'CrackBerry,' but the truth is our digital lifestyle truly can become habit-forming.**

priming you to be on the alert. In primal times, this response provided a direct benefit for safety and survival and, should things go horribly wrong, helped to manage pain. In *Are We Hardwired?: The Role of Genes in Human Behavior*, authors William R. Clark and Michael Grunstein discuss the role dopamine plays:

> It seems highly likely that stimulating dopamine release in the brain, which brings a sense of wellbeing, is also at play in altering the perception of pain. Wounded animals under attack use their opioids to set aside concern about pain in order to focus on escape.

With the demise of the saber-toothed tiger, so too ends our concern of being eaten alive by one. Yet the hardwiring for reacting and coping with such an event is still there. Today, it presents something like this: you hear the ding of a new text message, and the new stimulus diverts your attention. You get a little dopamine rush and it pulls you away from whatever you are doing for a quick glance. Then it happens again. And again. And yet again. With each ding, you receive a little jolt of addictive energy. Sure, we joke about the "CrackBerry," but the truth is our digital lifestyle truly can become habit-forming. Just ask MIT media scholar Judith Donath, who told *Scientific American* that digital rewards charge our compulsive behavior, and over time the effect becomes potent and hard to resist.

A 2012 *Newsweek* article entitled "Is the Web Driving Us Mad?" paints a more ominous picture. It states that constant digital use can actually shrink areas of the brain that are responsible for processing speech, memory, emotion, empathy, concentration, motor control, sensory information, and impulse control by up to twenty percent. Meanwhile, the brain experiences an increase of neurons receptive to speedy processing and instant gratification. Citing peer-reviewed research and neuroimagery scans showing brain similarities between digital addicts and drug addicts, the article proposed that the Internet may not only be making us dumber or lonelier, but also more depressed and anxious, prone to obsessive-compulsive and attention-deficit disorders.

> ❝ **It's comforting to know that air traffic controllers also take breaks every twenty minutes . . . for twenty minutes!** ❞

Clifford Nass, a communications professor at Stanford University, speculates that one sweeping cost of excess digital stimulation is diminished empathy—what psychologists believe to be one of the most profound defining characteristics of human relationships.[6] When the screen comes first, we often don't have or give enough time and energy to listen, absorb, and appreciate other people's feelings on an emotional level. Because young people tend to be in a constant mode of stimulation, they are particularly vulnerable.

In late 2010, *The New York Times* examined digital overstimulation in children in a front-page article called "Growing Up Digital, Wired for Distraction." Citing brain studies, the article states that periods of rest are critical for the brain to synthesize information, make connections between ideas, and develop a sense of self. It goes on to say that downtime is particularly important for young brains that have trouble focusing and setting priorities, ultimately recommending a digital diet. The experts who weighed in made the following suggestions: (1) balance screen time evenly between entertainment and educational activities, (2) eliminate multitasking options while studying, and (3) adults should act as a role model by setting an example of moderation.

MINI MENTAL BREAKS

Your brain does not operate in a linear manner like a cell phone battery going from fully charged to drained after a day of heavy use. Your brain craves stimulation and complex intellectual challenges, but it also needs to be frequently rested and refreshed. Scientists use the term *sustained attention* to describe the ability to focus and produce consistent results on a task over a period of time. One theory suggests that we are unable to sustain attention for longer than twenty minutes on any one thing. When we think we are sustaining attention longer, we are, in effect, repeatedly refocusing on the same thing. Obviously, it helps if we enjoy the activity, are competent at it, have high energy levels, and can operate in a low-stress, distraction-free environment.

But however much we may enjoy our work, we simply can't be productive 24/7! We require recovery from technology overload, and to some degree, our culture recognizes this. We've established customs that promote balance such as coffee breaks and lunch breaks during the workday, weekends to counter the workweek, and vacations away from our daily routines. The good intentions are there, but our brains need more. If you find yourself zoning out while engaged in an activity requiring sustained attention, it's a clear indication you need more breaks.

We can learn something from Las Vegas card dealers, who typically sustain intense on-the-job focus for forty minutes, followed by a twenty-minute break, and repeat this pattern throughout a shift. It's comforting to know that air traffic controllers also take breaks every twenty minutes . . . for twenty minutes! Construction workers and other physical laborers, too, are diligent about completely disengaging from the job at break time, removing gear, leaving the immediate area, and resting the brain. When the proverbial evening whistle blows, work ends punctually, no matter what's happening on the job site.

YOU ARE HARDWIRED *to be drawn to novel, potentially dangerous, details in your environment.*

MODERN DISCONNECT: *the next ding of an incoming text message.*

PRIMAL CONNECTION: *limited use of technology so it does not consume you.*

Contrast these positions with the typical office worker who disregards planned breaks or quitting times as the pressure to complete a project escalates. If you're working on a computer and your focus wavers, simply stop what you are doing, get up, and walk around for a minute or two. Focus your eyes on distant objects to ease the strain of sustained screen focus (or just close them for a bit), then return to the task at hand.

At least every two hours, take a longer break of five to ten minutes. The way you choose to unplug should be as dissimilar as possible to your work. Go outdoors and access fresh air, open space, and sunlight, and engage in some form of moderate physical activity. If your job is largely inactive, get up and move around over the course of an eight-hour workday as much as possible. Even five minutes of outdoor activity will oxygenate and energize your brain and body, making you more focused and productive when you return to your desk. If you experience a significant energy lull during the workday, try to fit in a twenty-minute nap to recharge.

After work, set boundaries. Remember Mister Rogers? Model him at the end of the day when you walk through the front door. Well, maybe not busting out your rendition of "Won't You Be My Neighbor?," but remove your coat and shoes, and change out of your work clothes into more comfortable attire. Put aside your digital gadgets, and allow yourself to completely decompress and immerse into a fresh environment of family, relaxation, and perhaps a hobby. Challenge yourself to disconnect. As a general rule, stay focused at work, but when you come home, stay tuned in there. Try not to skirt it with rationalizations as you fondle your iPhone in one hand, and push your child on the swing with the other.

MEDIA OBSESSION AND FRENETIC PASSIVITY

Before the invention of the printing press in 1440 AD, our context for experiencing current events was, relatively speaking, limited to the goings on within the clan, village, or settlement. Even as recently as the 1990s, before the Internet explosion, our nightly news was primarily national in its scope. Today, in the midst of the global and electronic media, we are each burdened with the fate of Atlas, under the weight of a world beset by incessant perils and calamities that can stretch our emotional dimensions beyond coping limits. In Grok's day,

MANAGE TECHNOLOGY WITH TECHNOLOGY

Customize and streamline your television viewing with a Digital Video Recorder (DVR). Choose the shows you want to watch, when you want to watch them, and fast-forward through commercials and other lulls. RSS feeds (Rich Site Summary) works in a similar fashion with your Internet content, basically taking the mass out of mass media. It works by compiling a "reader feed" with organized updates from all the sites to which you subscribe, and can be read in a short period of time. To create an account, go to Google.com/reader and follow the few simple steps. You can also check out other reputed RSS services, such as NetVibes, NetNewsWire, or Reeder for Apple. Look for the RSS icon—an orange square with white radio waves—on your favorite blogs, newspapers, and magazines. Click on the icon, and you become a subscriber. For your work commute, try downloading podcasts, books on tape, or customized song playlists on your iPod, or subscribe to satellite radio and enjoy commercial-free niche programming.

he could effectively act on the threats to his community and heal beyond its contained tragedies. In our day, the stakes are much higher and the implied community much broader.

Obviously, local, national, and global awareness is pretty much mandatory in order to be an informed and conscientious citizen these days. But, in your efforts to reclaim peace of mind, you would be well advised to find a healthy middle ground between immersing yourself in a constant barrage of bad news and dark emotions, and sticking your head in the sand. C. John Sommerville, author of *How the News Makes Us Dumb: The Death of Wisdom in an Information Society*, notes that our constant exposure to endless threads of instantaneous, disassociated "news" without the natural filters of time and context has the power to leave us overwhelmed and yet still lacking in the event's larger perspective. We'd do better, he suggests, spending less time staying on top of each trivial update and devoting more time to discussing, reflecting, and thoughtfully acting on the issues in which we feel most personally invested.

Heeding this advice requires realigning your perspective. You have a right, and a responsibility, to respect your emotional limits. The relative peace of this moment for one person is as genuine and meaningful as the tragedy befalling another. The world, we must remember, is more than the sum of its crises. Psychotherapist Miriam Greenspan spells this out in her book *Healing Through the Dark Emotions: The Wisdom of Grief, Fear, and Despair,* suggesting that we need to make peace with the "inevitable pain of being alive and being humanly connected to others." Nonetheless, she explains, we must also bring a protective consciousness to our interactions with the world, "cultivating a deep awareness of emotions as in-the-body energies, and of the thoughts that both trigger and subdue them."

One study of a hundred news broadcasts over a six-month period determined that over *half of all stories and total airtime* are characterized as VCS programming—an acronym for violence, conflict, and suffering.[7] Now, consider that a number of studies show a correlation between viewing disturbing news coverage and experiencing symptoms of post-traumatic stress disorder, as severe as if you had endured the event personally. This is no doubt the inevitable outcome of twenty-four-hour news channels that cycle the same stories all day long. One compelling study suggests that watching these events and feeling the anguish of those who are directly experiencing the impact can create feelings of anger, fear, and helplessness.[8]

Of course, information that you can actually impact, or could involve you, is vastly more important than random news you have no control over. Paris Hilton and Lindsay Lohan already have their own legal advisors. And while he seems to be far more reasonable and communicative than his father, the North Korean "supreme leader" Kim Jong-un is not likely to take your call any time soon, either. Ya know what I'm sayin'? To determine the appropriate level of your involvement with the news, ask yourself a few questions:

Can I take action and make an impact? Often we obsess more about global nuclear threats than about real suffering inside of our own social circles. If you get wind of strife involving someone you know, reach out and communicate with that person. Show your friend or family member that you care and are willing to help in any way possible. Yes, families deserve space and peace during difficult times, but I believe we use this as a cop-out to avoid uncomfortable communication. You have little to lose by reaching out and offering support—in general, becoming involved in the story.

What do I need to know? A major global event such as 9/11 beckons you to become informed on a deeper level. Major wars, terrorism, and catastrophes have a profound impact on the way we operate as a global society. Sorting through your thoughts and feelings with your family and friends is a way to strengthen these relationship bonds, help manage grief, and generally help make sense of the world.

Is there a lesson of value to absorb? The 1992 Los Angeles Riots, triggered by the "not guilty" Rodney King verdict, hit me hard because the graphic images dominating the evening news were in my hometown. Furthermore, the riots had national significance because they symbolized hot buttons of race relations, police brutality, and controversial jury verdicts. The images of mayhem were indeed salacious, but it was important for every single resident of Los Angeles— and across America—to understand the entire story and ponder carefully how we can "all just get along."

BECOME A BRUTALLY DEMANDING EDITOR

If you were to shine a light on the way you spend your time, what do you think you might find? One area I recommend taking a closer look at is how much time you devote to gathering information. How much of that precious time can you reclaim for more pleasurable pursuits? What would your day look like if you became a brutally demanding editor and filtered the stream of information that you allow into your world?

Some time ago, I devised a ten-minute drill where I limit myself to focused news and entertainment exposure at the beginning, and again at the end, of my workday. I was fascinated to discover how much high-priority information I could consume in such a seemingly short period. I obtained in those ten minutes more than enough information and diversion to keep me satiated throughout the day, and could comfortably disengage from events not related to my work until the next drill in the evening (again lasting around ten minutes). I had to catch myself a few times during the day, when my focus wandered and I noticed a habitual urge to click to a favorite news or entertainment bookmark. However, the discipline I exerted heightened the pleasure of my information feast in the evening.

One morning, I recorded the duration and specifics of the information I consumed and asked a close friend to do the same. My friend's experience revealed just how compelling the pull of distraction can be—even when he knew someone was keeping score! Let's take a look.

MARK'S NEWS AND ENTERTAINMENT BREAKDOWN

MarksDailyApple.com: Read a long-ish guest post (1,322 words) in its final edited form as well as the reader comments.

DrudgeReport.com: Read short article on national health care legislation (355 words).

HuffingtonPost.com: Read three articles (from Business, Media, and Healthy Living sections) totaling 1,700 words.

Weather.com: Read about a hurricane closing in on the Caribbean (262 words).

LetThemEatMeat.com: Skimmed a lengthy interview with an ex-vegan, by Denise Minger (6,300 words).

ESPN.com: Read article about NBA player trades (565 words).

Elapsed time: 12 minutes, 41 seconds

FRIEND'S NEWS AND ENTERTAINMENT BREAKDOWN

Local community newspaper: Read letter to editor (280 words) and comments. Read sports story on local high school athlete (560 words). Read sex scandal story about local business executive (387 words).

LATimes.com: Read a Sports/Business feature about the LA Dodgers's owner being heavily in debt (2,003 words). Read about the drug bust of Rapper T.I. (280 words; eyes wandered to headline/photo; wasted about 30 seconds).

TMZ.com Celebrity Gossip: Read about Paris Hilton's drug bust (297 words). Read article about Axl Rose's concert riot and lawsuit against his former manager (247 words).

MarksDailyApple.com: Read daily post about arthritis (1,617 words) and emailed link to two people with short note.

ZenHabits.com: Read post on "creating stillness" (709 words) and emailed a link to a friend with a short note.

Elapsed Time: 13 minutes, 26 seconds

Following the exercise, my friend sent along these comments:

I'm kind of embarrassed to send this, Mark. I mean, *TMZ.com Celebrity Gossip*? I couldn't care less about Paris Hilton and her cocaine purse, which she says isn't really her purse (but looks exactly like one she's holding in a photo she uploaded to Twitter a month prior, with the comment: 'Love my new Chanel purse'). A click took me there—I can't even remember where I started from—and it honestly took a couple minutes for me to escape from the grips of the 'excess digital stimulation,' as you say.

The Los Angeles Times story about the debt problems of Dodgers owner Frank McCourt turned out to be a super long article. I didn't even care that much and sped through pretty quickly, but I simply wasn't disciplined enough to fold my cards halfway through the piece. Another waste of time. I also noticed just how salacious and lowbrow even my local community newspaper is. I couldn't help but finish the executive sex scandal story. I reflected on the previous week of headlines in this local community newspaper—all relating to crime, sex, violence, or just shenanigans—and promptly canceled the subscription I've held for more than twenty years. I tried the ten-minute drill again that evening and did much better. In eight minutes, I read stories that were entertaining and meaningful and caught up on all the day's news, which I ignored per your request without much difficulty during the workday.

When it's time to open the floodgates of email, voicemail, Facebook, forum posting, web browsing, or digital entertainment options, keep your editor's hat on. Filter quickly through less important communication and either ignore or offer brief responses. When my friend Timothy Ferris—author of *The Four-Hour Work Week: Escape 9-5, Live Anywhere and Join the New Rich*—sends me email, it's always brief, with an disclaimer under his signature line:

YOU ARE HARDWIRED *to solve problems and be creative.*

MODERN DISCONNECT: *associating quantity with quality.*

PRIMAL CONNECTION: *take frequent breaks to refresh your brain.*

Q: Why is this email five sentences or less?
A: http://five.sentenc.es

The link takes you to a very short explanation of how emails are often too lengthy to respond to, resulting in continuous inbox overflow for those who receive a lot of it. The answer? Treat all email responses like text messages, using short sentences that cut to the chase. It's ingenious, really. Such responses respect your time as well as the recipient's.

If you agree that time is one of our greatest assets, choose very carefully who and what is allowed even a tiny nugget of yours. Occasionally watching a YouTube video recommended by a friend only takes a few minutes, and it might even make your day—unfortunately, that can't be said for every email joke, chain letter, or request that comes your way. And on some occasions, settling into an engaging blog, casually browsing iTunes for new songs, or researching something of interest can be considered quality leisure time. What I'm talking about here is disconnecting from the continual stream of information throughout your day and tightening and narrowing that time into a shorter window.

MINDLESS MULTITASKING VS. MINDFUL SINGLE-TASKING

As the efficiency and convenience of technology continues to escalate, there is a strong temptation to multitask in order to keep pace with hectic modern life. Multitasking has even become a buzzword in job postings—a desirable prerequisite skill for employment candidates. Witness the typical office worker, who in an average hour switches to a different working window on his or her computer screen nearly thirty-seven times! That's in addition to getting distracted every three minutes with emails, phone calls, the Internet, and other interruptions.

Of course, this constant back and forth makes for a rather disjointed existence. That, researchers say, is the real concern. Met with constant interruption, our thinking becomes scattered and jumbled. At times, we can feel like we're playing multiple shell games, trying to recall where we were in the midst of each one. Researchers tell us that the persistent intrusions and diversions of this technological multitasking leave our brains fatigued. A Stanford University study showed that media multitaskers are unable to pay attention, control their memory, or switch from one job to another as well as those who prefer to complete one task at a time. In other words, they have a harder time filtering out the irrelevant from the relevant, resulting in the counterproductive effect of slowing them down.

When faced with a deluge of digital information and a lack of downtime to synthesize it intellectually, reflect on it, and make meaning of it, we tax our working memory. Studies have also shown that multitasking compromises learning and impairs memory recall. And this is not just in the work environment. By design, television programs pack in large amounts of information in short bursts, presenting a roller coaster of staccato dialogue, crash-and-burn scenes, and fast-moving images that change every three to four seconds. Moreover, Internet users spend an average of less than a minute on any given website, browsing fast and furiously, completely changing the stimulus with the click of a button. As for text messaging, teenagers are apt to do it all day long, simultaneously carrying on multiple abbreviated "conversations" at a given time.[9]

Maybe Grok was a bit of a multitasker, too. He's walking down the path, he's in search of berries, in search of prey, and on the lookout for predators. He's

SO YOU HAVE A SPASTIC IMAGINATION...

Impulsive thoughts often lead to creative ideas. If your mind wanders in a creative direction while working on another project, I recommend taking notes about these streams of consciousness for later access. Go ahead and welcome your impulses and tangents, but understand that there is a clear distinction between creative impulses that randomly originate in your own mind and the buzzing of a text message breaking your train of thought. Take the necessary preventive measures against digital interlopers, however, and power down or unplug entirely. When a creative thought flies into your mind, go with the flow, take some notes if you need to, then gently return your focus to the task at hand.

looking at the broken twigs, he's smelling the breeze, maybe picking up whiffs of scat. The difference, however, is that he is exercising habit #4 (be here now), and is completely in the present moment. He is keenly aware of his surroundings, comprised of variables that all have a relationship to the here and now—unlike the accountant with the phone shouldered against his ear discussing dinner plans with his wife while updating last quarter's financial spreadsheet.

Neuroscientist Gary Aston-Jones of the Medical University of South Carolina theorizes that the more you increase your level of multitasking, the more you potentially harm your ability to do tasks that require intense sustained focus other tasks such as writing, creating art, or performing scientific and mathematical equations.[10] What's more, there is evidence to support that multitaskers aren't even good at multitasking! MIT neuroscience professor Earl Miller says that we cannot truly multitask, because our brains can only process a single stream of information at a time.[11] When we say we are multitasking, we are actually just switching back and forth between tasks with amazing speed, creating the illusion of doing many things at once.

Even worse is multitasking while operating machinery. Seems pretty darn obvious, doesn't it? But a widely reported study from the Virginia Department of Transportation has found that texting while driving is twenty-three times more likely to result in an accident than driving while paying full attention to the road. Unfortunately, the pull of digital stimulation—chasing that damn

PERSONAL EXPERIMENT: TRY A TECHNOLOGY FAST

For one day, see if you can survive without your car, TV, computer, or other technology. Bicycle to the farmers market and bring home some bounty in your backpack or basket. Work your way leisurely through the Sunday paper, the accumulating magazine pile, or that page-turner gathering dust on your night table. When it gets dark, light a few candles and break out the board games—and that vintage bottle of red wine you've been saving for a special occasion.

high, again—is so strong that 81 percent of drivers admit to cell phone use while driving and 21 percent admit to texting, an activity six times more lethal than drunk driving. Even with sobering stories (such as celebrity plastic surgeon Dr. Frank Ryan fatally driving off the edge of Pacific Coast Highway in Malibu in 2010, reportedly distracted by texting), we continue to succumb to distraction and make stupid mistakes.

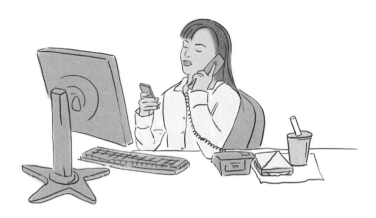

ZONE IN AND ZEN OUT

You can probably relate to the blissful feeling of being "in the zone," totally consumed by the moment as you pursue a challenging task. You're in a timeless space where your cerebellum—your primal, reactive, sensory brain—synergizes with the concentrated feedback delivered by your neocortex. This is "bottom up" processing, a melding of reasoning and sensing together. You experience this mode when you start sinking putts effortlessly after months of tedious technique lessons directed to your "top down" processing. It's when you step up and roll three strikes in a row at the company bowling outing after not touching a ball for decades. Here, your neocortex is certainly engaged—sticking your fingers into the ball, approaching the pins and pendulum swinging your arms—but zone experiences like these go beyond mere correct mechanics to access a higher state of functioning.

Writers, composers, and artists are intimately aware of the great gifts a focused and integrated mind can produce. They're also familiar with how elusive it can be. Legendary novelist, playwright, and screenwriter William Goldman (*Butch Cassidy and the Sundance Kid, All the President's Men, The Princess Bride, The Stepford Wives,* and many others) was asked in an interview about his formula for success, to which came his deadpan reply: "Get up very early in the morning and work very, very hard." A photo accompanying the interview shows Goldman in his cramped New York City office, featuring a tattered folding metal chair and a simple desk, a most unlikely command center for one of America's most successful writers. Goldman explained that he didn't want to create too comfortable a working environment for fear of distraction!

With some devoted effort, you can become adept at focusing on a single task at a time, too. First, flex your focusing muscles on some easy stuff. Zen out while chopping vegetables, raking leaves, walking the dog, or talking on the phone. Zero in on the flavors you taste in a glass of wine, your morning cup of joe, the sound of a fan, a reflection in a window, and let the rest of the world dissolve into the peripheral pool. The trick is to turn off your internal autopilot and stay completely present through a succession of mundane activities. Single-tasking, you'll discover, creates space to appreciate nuanced details and find beauty in the moment.

You will begin to see more clearly just how often artificial stimuli can add extra layers of distraction to your daily routine, and how removing those layers for periods of time can make you feel more calm. This is not to say you must sit idly on subway rides home instead of catching up on work or entertainment via mobile technology. What I'm suggesting here is that you notice how your day plays out differently when you carefully manage external stimuli and focus on the moment. At least once a day, try to keep your focusing muscles toned by slowing your pace and single-tasking on a succession of mundane endeavors. By being present for the typically autopiloted activities from time to time, you will fine-tune your focusing powers for your more intellectually complex challenges. At the end of the day, concentrated focus is something to cultivate throughout our lives and something that, in turn, cultivates us.

Silence is a true friend who never betrays.
CONFUCIUS

SLOWING DOWN

TORTOISE OR HARE, YOU DECIDE. Who do you want to be? Why not a little bit of both? With the ebb and flow of our energy output and the assumption that we exist in an age of efficiency, we tend to think and move *fast, fast, fast*. We tend to live more like the hare than the tortoise. To our sympathetic nervous system, our current-day lifestyle is a near-opposite image to that of our hunter-gatherer ancestors, who lived more like the tortoise, moving at a slow pace occasionally interrupted by brief moments of terror. Contrast that to our frenetic lives interspersed with fleeting glimpses of calm. Indeed, we all to some degree live with our society's obsession with speed. Whether it's with omnipresent traffic, constant deadlines, or crammed schedules, too many of us spend too much time running or being overrun.

In the cursory sweeps of our day, we miss out on the nuanced textures of life—the sensory pleasures of a good meal, the subtle changes in our growing child's face, the quiet beauty of a weekend morning, the warm connection with a partner or friend. What do we do when we find ourselves caught in an unsustainable

YOU ARE HARDWIRED *to live life at a slow pace.*

MODERN DISCONNECT: *society's obsession with speed.*

PRIMAL CONNECTION: *practicing rhythm, ritual, and flow.*

momentum? Some have found the answer in a growing international movement known as Slow Living, an offshoot of the Slow Food movement that began in Italy during the 1980s with a call to return to the basics and to support the personal and social pleasures of eating.

One of the central voices of the Slow Living movement, Carl Honoré, argues our society is caught in an ever-escalating "arms race" of speed. In one of the movement's seminal books, *In Praise of Slowness: How a Worldwide Movement Is Challenging the Cult of Speed*, Honoré illuminates a sad reality shaped by everything from fast food to "one-minute bedtime stories" as well as research on workers who face burnout in their twenties and thirties, and doctors whose minimal time with patients causes them to miss pertinent, if not critical, information. Our addiction to speed, Honoré warns, is undermining our personal relationships, our societal civility, our individual fulfillment, and our physical health.

Speed in this sense is more than a velocity, as Slow Living proponents explain. It morphs sooner or later into a personal and collective mindset. It becomes the rationalization behind all manner of pernicious choices. From a societal standpoint, for example, it could be that relying on "fast" farming methods—such as concentrated animal feeding operations and genetically modified organisms— produces short-term profits with long-term consequences. On a personal level, it can encompass all of the games we play with ourselves to stay above water, like eating grab-on-the-run foods, neglecting fitness and play, using stimulants to get

A SPACE OF ONE'S OWN

Find a space in your house (or backyard). It could be as big as a small room or as small as a windowsill. Do whatever needs doing to preserve that area against clutter, small children, and other intruders. Claim it as your personal space for reading, meditation, or just a few minutes of quiet alone time each day. Put whatever you want there: a pillow or chair, a candle, worry beads, a plant, your grandfather's pocket watch, or absolutely nothing at all. If it's a windowsill, put something interesting outside of it: a bird feeder, a suncatcher, some foliage. Go there. Every day—at least once.

> **Slow living—in all its spheres—seeks, above all, to cultivate reflection and appreciation.**

through another afternoon, giving up sleep, and multitasking our way through each day. In our attempts to meet the most immediate obligations, we miss filling our most essential needs.

Beyond the logistical strategies and short-term fixes, there's a better way: bring attention to all spheres of life. It's about living one's values and giving our time and attention accordingly. Experience tells us that slow activities and a slower pace make for a more relaxing experience. People everywhere take up "slow hobbies" like knitting or woodcarving. We enjoy the quieting influence of an ambling stroll at night. We relish the slow and sensory feast of a big holiday dinner.

Yet, there's science to support the call to decelerate. Long, slow, low-level aerobic workouts, for example, are correlated with everything from increased longevity to reduced risk of metabolic syndrome, breast cancer, and cardiovascular disease.[12] "Slow agriculture"—the act of raising livestock with biologically appropriate feeds such as grass grazing and growing crops without the use of the synthetic pesticides—makes for a more enriching and nourishing (and less toxic) food supply. Activities that induce the quiet state of mental flow can ease symptoms of anxiety and challenge us in positive, healthful ways.

Living slowly ultimately means living deeply. Slow travel, for example, is both a lesson in its own right and a metaphor for the movement. There's something missed in hitting just the postcard sites of a city we travel to and then moving on to the next destination. We have the photo memento for our collection, but we return home relatively unchanged. Committing to a single destination for as long a time as our vacation allows us the chance to delve into the culture of a place— to experience the subtler but more telling characteristics of a locale. We meet the people, hear the stories, feel the communal rhythm. With time and attention, we encounter a place and let its influence permeate us. We return home different, richer for the journey.

This example highlights the importance of incubation, that rich period in which the influence of an experience synthesizes with self. Time and mental space is critical for this absorption. Slow living—in all its spheres—seeks, above all, to cultivate reflection and appreciation. It calls us to commit our time and passion to what feels most natural and life giving.

How do I see the connection between Slow Living and Primal living? I think Slow Living on some level reclaims what is natural in human relations, basic sustenance, and life balance. More than that, however, I like how Slow Living in many respects brings us closer to some of our evolutionary patterns. Sure, Grok wasn't pondering the virtues of a "slow" stock portfolio or holding workshops on tantric sex (although who knows?). Nonetheless, the core of the movement rings true—and timeless. There's a reason we miss quiet weekends untethered to technology. There's a reason a city with ample park space and a vibrant pedestrian zone feels more inviting than a congested sea of skyscrapers and cars. There's a reason we feel uniquely fulfilled cooking and sharing a homemade meal with others. These were the basic experiences of our ancestors. Humanity evolved with rhythms and rituals that modern acceleration has left in the dust. Our psyches haven't caught up with the change of pace. Life makes more sense the slow way.

THE RHYTHM OF RITUAL

Perhaps meditation is the antidote, or at least part of the slowing-down solution. There are some who argue meditation is just another modern exercise. I say it's one of the not-so-modern inventions that help us live well in the modern age—a principle inherent to the Primal Connection. We can trace the idea back to rituals, one of the earliest steps in our social evolution.

When we talk about ritual today, we think of collective traditions like holiday customs or religious conventions. But rituals in their clear, patterned ease can serve as touchstones for our intention to stay in the moment or to cultivate relaxation during the day. Whether it is a certain succession of activities before bedtime or a yoga practice in the morning, these rituals can produce substantial effects on our wellbeing.

In some regard, of course, a ritual can be any repeated activity to which we bring a positive and intentional mindfulness. As Julia Cameron puts it in *The Artist's Way: A Spiritual Path to Higher Creativity*, the brain is reached through rhythm, not reason. Certainly you've experienced this phenomenon, and perhaps not paid much attention to it. Some people like the rhythm of walking. Others engage in pampering rituals or take special care in meaningful hobbies, like the careful laying out of tools in preparation for woodcarving or the setup of paints and canvas for painting. Although we might not be thinking of it at the time, even ritual in this alternative sense may connect us to some bigger association or emotional story. Maybe you're laying out the tools like your father did. Maybe setting up the painting supplies this way is a kind of homage to the well of creativity you hope to tap. Our efforts don't have to be big or bold to contain an element of ceremony.

Beyond any sense of reverence, the simple act of repetition can somehow act as a meditation and invoke positive feelings. Researchers have shown that simple routine enhances feelings of safety, confidence, and wellbeing. Go ahead and do ten sun salutations (yes, right now) and see how you feel.[13] More relaxed? Of course you are. For millennia, repetitive movements such as yoga have played a role in ritual—and are as old as human society itself.

Think about the rituals that populate your life right now. Maybe you don't refer to them as rituals, but include any routine that's somehow calming, that helps you mindfully transition from one part of your day to the next. Put them under the light of assessment if that makes sense. Which are comforting, life-giving, or otherwise positive influences? Which, if any, have lost their core of meaning and now just take up mental and logistical space in hollow forms? Is it time for redefining old rituals or creating new ones?

ONE WITH THE WORLD

Flow follows rhythm and ritual. But it isn't something we find, as if it can be rationally sought out. On the contrary, it comes to us when we finally release that hold on reason and intent. Flow moments happen when we become wholly absorbed in our endeavors. They are sometimes called peak performances or "in the zone" moments in the athletic arena. Flow happens when we let consciousness—or self-consciousness—slip away in a larger pursuit. We can experience it when skiing down a mountain, climbing the face of a rocky cliff, playing Frisbee with the kids, rowing across a quiet lake, creating music or art, practicing yoga, or building a cabinet. We can encounter it either in an individual activity or as part of a collective group. Under the spell of flow, we become our action, our intent, our doing.

They're moments when the rest of the world—even awareness itself—recedes into an unperceived periphery. Seemingly outside the progression of time, detached from the bounds of physical need, you fade past existence into immersion. The self quietly falls away. You're one with the mountain, the paintbrush, the instrument, the pose, the stride, the notes, the words. If you could freeze time to capture this Dasein experience, you'd witness freedom, lightness, unwitting joy. (Dasein, by the way, is one of my favorite words, a German term meaning "being in the world.")

Like a faint star in the night sky, however, flow moments resist direct observation. The minute we bring attention to them, they've already passed. We catch them, instead, out of the corner of our eye—briefly, fleetingly, on the returning threshold of consciousness. Despite their transience, we discern their effects. We've lived those moments outside of time and thought. We've felt, we've sensed, we've intuited. Inevitably, we emerge changed—more content, composed.

The father of flow research is Mihaly Csikszentmihalyi, a Hungarian professor and researcher. His research and analysis of flow experiences have been applied to everything from educational theory to business management. Csikszentmihalyi's basic premise is this: we most enjoy life when we're presented with—or seek out—manageable but creative challenges that tap into our individual curiosities and interests, challenges that give us immediate feedback for our improvement and success. They're enough to stimulate our biochemical triggers without setting off the whole fight-or-flight cascade. These constructive trials of choice and circumstance offer a stark contrast to the getting and spending, passive entertainment, and personal pampering modern society often promotes as self-fulfillment. Csikszentmihalyi says it best:

> When a person's entire being is stretched in the full functioning of body and mind, whatever one does becomes worth doing for its own sake; living becomes its own justification. In the harmonious focusing of physical and psychic energy, life finally comes into its own. It is the full involvement of flow, rather than happiness, that makes for excellence in life.[14]

In short, a life marked by flow has the power of "good" stress, of healthy, nurturing challenge that feeds our sense of self-purpose as well as our self-affirmation. At the hectic pace of modern life, with its disjointed rhythms and constant interruptions, it's easy to become distanced from these states of flow. In the process, I believe, we become distanced from ourselves. When we allow ourselves to think about it, we can feel on the fringe, outside of life looking in, pining to return to the center. (Should we say life crisis?) Ennui, Csikszentmihalyi tells us, is the acute opposite of flow (a state few of us, I hope, experience). With ennui, we're somehow left with little but the self—detached from the indivisible human context of purpose, action, community.

Although most of us probably wouldn't put ourselves in that most discouraging category, we all now and then can lose touch with transcendence in our lives. We "forget" how to slip into these flow states. Some 20 percent of participants in one study reported flow experiences each day, but another 15 percent said they never felt them.[15] Research suggests, however, that we can, indeed, train ourselves to get back in the groove. As Csikszentmihalyi explains, "One of the most important active ingredients here is the refinement of attention. . . . Training attention to come back over and over again to a complex task allows awareness to become increasingly absorbed in the task at hand."[16]

In one study, professional musicians who received yoga training for a summer reported less performance anxiety than those in a control group who did not train with yoga. In a subsequent study, musicians who participated in an ongoing yoga program experienced less self-consciousness during performances and reported an easier time slipping into flow states, or *autotelic* states (having a purpose in and not apart from itself).[17]

We all, I believe, have that craving for transcendence in our lives. There are days when we feel the weight of our self-consciousness as a burden. As I've mentioned before, we're a curious, high-maintenance species, yet still a fascinating lot. A healthy life with all the wholesome trimmings— nourishing food, vigorous exercise, adequate sleep— indeed does us well. But there's a major divide separating surviving versus thriving.

YOU ARE HARDWIRED *to engage in silence and reflection.*

MODERN DISCONNECT: *busyness, noise pollution, and crammed schedules.*

PRIMAL CONNECTION: *solo retreats and escapes.*

GOING FAST ... AT A LEISURELY PACE

In the late 1980s, I coached a team of world-ranked professional triathletes. It was interesting to observe and compare the difference in their training routines with the amateurs I had trained with in previous years. The typical amateur triathlete was a type-A overachiever with a demanding career and a busy family life. Fitting in the requisite workouts was a constant juggling act between work and family obligations. The word "squeeze" was used repeatedly to describe scheduling efforts, starting with the morning alarm and an abrupt commencement of the day's first workout. Pacing seemed to be an obsession, not just for tracking workout speed, but minding the clock at all times in order to remain "on time" for every item on the packed daily agenda. The popular "quick lunchtime swim workout" referred more to the peripherals than the lap times—rushing out of the office, a presto change-o in the locker room, a one-minute post-workout shower, and then bursting back into the office an hour later with water beads still dripping from hair onto collar.

In contrast, the professional athletes—whose job was simply to race fast—lived lives centered around their workouts, with minimal interference from real-life distractions or social obligations. While the pros conducted their workouts aggressively, the pace of their lives was leisurely. Lunchtime swim? Sure, but instead of toweling off, jerking the tie back into place and rushing out to the parking lot, the post-swim routine for the pros consisted of lingering in the poolside spa for nearly as long as the workout, shooting the breeze, stretching tight muscles, and generally decompressing from the intense effort in the water. Eventually, the pack moved from the spa into an easy lunch involving more shooting of the breeze. Eventually, they remounted their bikes for a couple more hours of pedaling, then took an afternoon nap, followed by a late-day run, followed by a stretching/icing session, followed by a quiet evening of television, reading, or lingering over a huge meal. As I spent more time in their world, I learned that the competitive advantage enjoyed by these professionals went beyond their impressive workouts. Embracing life both with purpose and at a more leisurely pace produces extraordinary results.

It behooved our ancestors to push themselves beyond mere subsistence living. Instinctive, adaptive curiosity was likely the mother of invention more than a preconceived notion of necessity. How do we feed that instinct today? How do we honor the need for concentration and competence? How do we lose ourselves to achieve that contentment and quiet center?

In the busyness of life, it can be hard to carve out time and focus, but perhaps our ability to experience flow depends less on separate efforts than on a mindset and organization we bring to many of those daily demands—work, hobbies, or fitness-related endeavors. Flow isn't about doing a particular thing as much as it is about losing ourselves in it. The rhythm of snow shoveling (yes, even that with a little imagination), the creative inspiration of cooking, the abandon of

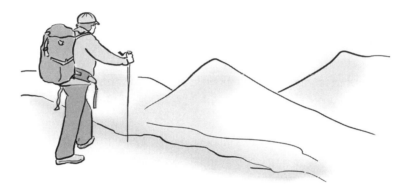

a good hike or run, the precision or inventiveness of our work can all become fodder for flow. When we let go of the extraneous commentary in our heads, the resentment of the task at hand, the impatience with ourselves, we can bring a new engagement to the moment—and in the process find ourselves altered as a result.

AS I PONDER'D IN SILENCE

As is often the case with questions of health, the real issue isn't just what to avoid but what to embrace. Take silence, for example. Is it just the absence of noise, or is there something deeper that defines silence—something we'd do well to understand, contemplate, or invite into our lives?

Author George Prochnik explains it well in his book *In Pursuit of Silence*: "The loudest argument for quiet may be a reflection on what otherwise remains in danger of going unheard." What is it that we're listening for? What are we hoping to apprehend or appreciate when we peel away the layers of noise from our lives? For each of us, perhaps, a different answer may come to mind.

From my own perspective, understanding silence has increasingly been an attempt toward grounding these last few years, a burrowing deep into what I've come to identify as a primal, or as certain thinkers have described it, elemental levels of consciousness and subconsciousness. Silence isn't just an effort toward relaxation or an escape from modern layers of busyness but a reconnection in some regard with what is most natural and most essential to our still-present primal selves.

In *Original Wisdom: Stories from an Ancient Way of Knowing*, Robert Wolff writes about the "overload" of our modern environments. He offers, "I am certain I am not the only one who has to turn off some senses in a supermarket or in a train station or in an airport…. One learns—has to learn—to shut off some senses, to protect oneself from all that noise." Sound familiar?

For me, striving toward silence has been two things. It's been about spending as much time as possible in environments that don't necessitate a deadening of the senses. Yet, it has also largely been an attempt to shut off the mental chatter, to forget putting words to anything altogether for a few minutes. Truth be told, I have a hard time banishing all thought and releasing all perception. Better for me, I've found, not to shut out the scenery but to slip into it, to more fully attend to and apprehend what's around me (the simpler and more natural the surroundings the better) without words but with the senses. In this regard, silence for me has become less an introversion or escape than an individually measured, deliberate approaching of where I'm at.

In my silent mode, I see problems and goals from a different angle— something difficult to achieve, try as I might, when I'm grinding away in the office. I'm talking about poring over numerous drafts of a book cover, knowing we haven't nailed it yet, but not knowing exactly what's missing. Then, coming home from a muddy hike, not having spoken a word or thought about the book cover in three hours, a different vision will pop into my head as I'm hosing off my feet in the driveway. Sure enough, this will end up being the winning cover image. All that hard work, back-and-forth group emailing, and paralysis by analysis, when what I really needed was some silent downtime and muddy feet!

"They lived in small bands, roamed expanses of land, and engaged in traditions such as vision quests."

You can probably relate to experiencing a refreshing new perspective or a random epiphany in conjunction with a retreat of some form. What's going on here? In *A Book of Silence*, author Sara Maitland explains that silence connects you to the prelinguistic, prelogical "seedbed of self." Language is seated in a different part of the brain—the cerebral cortex—than all other vocalizations such as laughing, crying, shouting, which are controlled subcortically. When you let go of rational linguistic responses—the wearing conversations that go on both inside your head and with other people all day long— Maitland proposes that you can attune yourself to alternative, less intellectual, but raw, deeper levels of emotional experience. This solo, silent portal to a deeper emotional experience is clearly a component of our genetic makeup that supports creativity, problem solving, and peace of mind.

As evidenced by anthropological findings and the lifestyle patterns of traditional hunter-gatherer societies, our ancestors indulged in plenty of solitude during both daily tasks and leisure time. They lived in small bands, roamed expanses of land, and engaged in traditions such as vision quests— personal, spiritual retreats into the wilderness, often involving fasting—that served (and still do) as a rite of passage for the Native American Inuits and other indigenous cultures. Time away from the tribe allowed individuals to improve self-sufficiency, return to the group stronger, wiser, and with more to offer as a result of the seclusion.

A 2011 article in *The New York Times* called "Getting Far, Far Away From It All" details the influence of silent, solo retreats on high-powered, overworked professionals. This is serious stuff, with participants heading off to remote meditation centers and ceasing contact with other humans and the outside world for anywhere from a week to a month. During these lerungs—as they are called in Tibetan Buddhism—participants are encouraged to spend their days meditating, reciting mantras, doing basic exercise and chores, thinking positively, reading Buddhist texts, journaling, and preparing meals.

"You learn what's healthy for you, what you want to accept into your life, and what you want to leave behind," said one participant featured in the article. "I very strongly identified who I wanted in my life and who I didn't want. I came back and took some action." Another participant, a New York ad executive, emerged from the month-long retreat "knowing that it was time to shut down the brick-and-mortar aspect" of his business. While proceeding through a series of seven separate month-long retreats, the executive transformed his agency into a home-based consulting shop and moved out of Manhattan to a Brooklyn neighborhood where he teaches yoga and meditation on the side. How's that for life changing?

The article points out that some participants "just flip" after their first day and bail. But can you appreciate the insights shared by these serious enthusiasts, and maybe tackle something a little more comfortable and bite-sized yourself?

In distancing yourself from everyday buzz and chatter, you may discover elements of yourself that have been long neglected. Consider this quote from novelist and opinion columnist Anna Quindlen: "The truth about your own life is not always easy to accept, and sometimes hasn't even occurred to you." I love this quote. But it also makes me feel a bit uneasy. I don't want to be that guy, oblivious to my own truths and too busy to bother with such matters. And when my life gets hectic and stressful, I realize that I am trending in that direction instead of toward enlightenment. At all times, you are only a few steps away from silence and solitude or, alternatively, from stress and tension. Take advantage of those opportunities, large and small.

Find time each day to be quiet and by yourself—even if just for a few minutes. Nature is the ideal setting, but if ten minutes in your car or a secluded area of your office is all you can manage, that's fine, too. I sometimes leave my office, and head outdoors for just a few minutes of silence. Hours later, it still has a significant impact on my disposition. Focus on getting into a routine with minimal difficulty. It isn't about the duration so much as it is about just doing it. Disengaging from everything, even for only a few minutes, suggests that you care enough about yourself to slow down and balance the perpetual busyness of daily life.

SECTION SUMMARY

Honoring the Sun: Falling asleep soon after dark and awakening to the rising of the sun has stamped our gene pattern for 2.5 million years. With the advent of electricity, we've managed to override this powerful circadian rhythm that not only governs sleep, but hunger, wakefulness, and hormones supporting health and wellbeing. Research suggests we have a natural preference for segmented sleep and our modern schedules—with long hours of wakefulness and shortened, single-sleep cycles—leave many of us sleep deprived. Take that nap, and your productivity will increase; it's a normal inclination in keeping with our biphasic sleep imprint. Make your bedroom a sanctuary for sleep, relaxation, and intimacy, in which you court refreshing sleep with silence and darkness. And avoid late-night lighting and digital stimulation.

Finding Focus: Most of us suffer from information overload, which in the last two decades has increased exponentially with global and electronic media, bringing us a barrage of bad news and dark emotions. The world, we must remember, is more than the sum of its crises. We need to protect our emotional limits by cultivating highly discriminating editorial skills. The brain craves stimulation and complex intellectual challenges but requires downtime as well. Work demands, distractions, and interruptions have us making mental jumps at an ever-increasing pace until we lose the ability to prioritize or we disconnect altogether. Differentiate your personal life from your work life and diligently power down at home, mentally as well as electronically. As for multitasking, the more you do, the more you harm your ability to sustain your focus. Turn off the autopilot and stay present while performing a single mundane task; you'll learn to carry this sort of focus over to peak performance tasks, even in a hectic environment.

Slowing Down: Our addiction to speed undermines personal relationships, societal civility, and individual fulfillment—not to mention physical health. Rhythmic rituals, such as yoga, help to restore a sense of calm and enhance positive and intentional mindfulness. A slower pace engages the brain and relieves stress and worry, inducing a state of relaxation—even flow. Flow moments happen when you become wholly absorbed in your endeavors. The rest of the world seems to recede to the edges of your awareness. Inevitably, you emerge more content and composed. By cultivating a healthy personal climate—nourishing food, vigorous exercise, adequate sleep—you find your ideal rhythm.

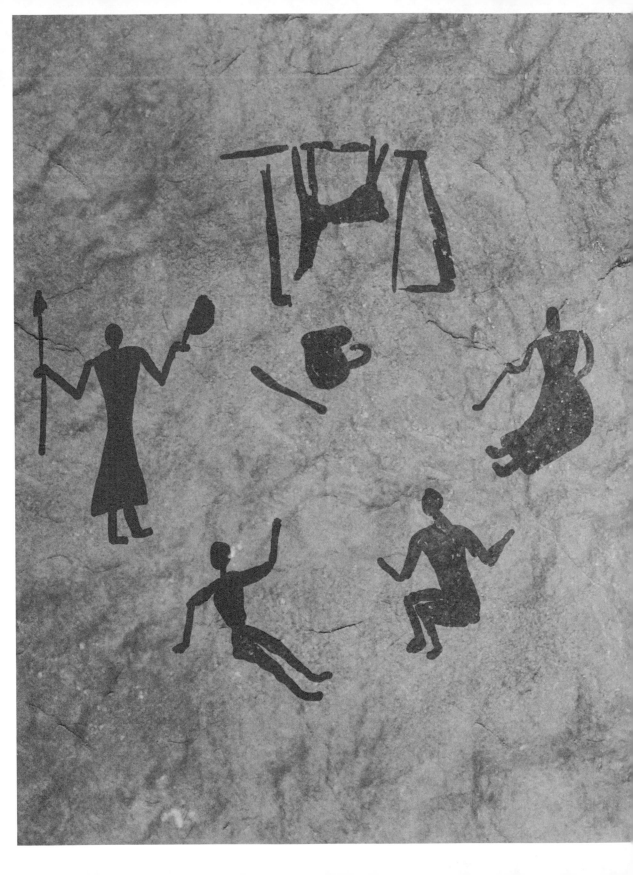

THE SOCIAL CONNECTION

HOW CAN WE ILLUMINATE OUR relationships with one another—those complicated, layered, critical, but confounding bonds we share? What's behind the sense of disconnect that so many of us feel today, and how can the ways of the hunter-gatherer help us reorient ourselves toward more fulfilling and resilient family circles and social connections? We evolved within the network of band communities, seeking out emotional and social bonds. That legacy continues to shape us today. The point, of course, is to reconnect with our original bearings and to restore the social orientations that are so critical to our human identity and wellbeing.

My father always used to say that when you die,
if you've got five real friends, then you've had a great life.

LEE IACOCCA

THE INNER CIRCLE

MANY SOCIAL BEHAVIORS WE BELIEVE are culturally learned are in fact hard-wired, established over several million years of survival. Indeed, those who formed strong social bonds were more likely to survive over the antisocial outliers, who, without the support of the clan, stood a higher risk of succumbing to a similar fate as the slow and the weak. Through tight social bonds, our ancestors relayed critical information to benefit the individual and the clan: where to get food, water, and shelter; what dangers to avoid; how to navigate vast territory on extended hunts or journeys; best techniques for hunting, gathering, or caring for children.

Research suggests that the social organization of hunter-gatherer bands supported a larger networking and member exchange with neighboring bands.[1] This arrangement both decreased violence (compared to other primates) and enhanced learning between groups. It most certainly kept the gene pool vital as well.

Bands generally ranged between twenty-five to fifty people in size, with looser ties on the periphery to perhaps some one hundred fifty or so (Typically a group of this size would form to increase the odds of survival, for example, hunkering down for the winter.)[2] Despite the extended contact, life revolved mainly around the intimacy of the inner circle, those few dozen adults and children who formed a kinship. Within the group there were typically enough hands to make hunting and foraging more productive, but not so many that disorganization took over.

Our ancestors' sense of self was pretty much wrapped up in how they supported the clan, and how they were accepted and supported by it. However, anthropologists point out that hunter-gatherer affiliation didn't absorb individuals into a subsumed "school of fish" identity, either.[3] They formed individual personalities that did not prove themselves by detachment but unfolded within supportive relationships.

The intimacy of the tribe would ultimately take shape not just in how well members collaborated in a day's work, but how they participated together in a night's cultural life, the emblem of which was the fire circle. With ample leisure time and the obvious motivation to stay with the group in the dark hours of night, tribe members shared stories and song. They danced and celebrated. They shared in and passed on cosmologies that reflected a mystical narrative of life in their region as well as accounts of ancestors who came before them.

The fire circle, suggests Paul Shepard, author of *Coming Home to the Pleistocene*, is a vivid metaphor for the intimacy of hunter-gatherer socialization and small-scale human affairs. Not only does the fire circle reflect the basic social structure with which we evolved, but also the sustaining social and cultural activities—everything from story to ceremony, feast to music—that nurtured human ties. The fire circle encompassed communal participation, shared ritual, and kinship investment. It's a poignant Primal metaphor for reconnecting with a deeper, more fulfilling social experience of the world.

FRIENDS WITH HEALTH BENEFITS

What comes to mind when you think of your friends? The reading club, Tuesday card games, progressive dinners, Saturday morning golf, and summer barbecues? The talks over coffee, cocktails, racquetball, quilting, dog walking, or maybe just over the phone? Friends, new and old, close and far-flung, hold a special place in our sentiments. We value the history we have with

YOU ARE HARDWIRED *for meaningful personal connections.*

MODERN DISCONNECT: *virtual relationships displacing actual relationships.*

PRIMAL CONNECTION: *replace Facebook time with face-to-face time.*

them, the perspective they bring, the support they offer, the stories they tell, the interests we share. Without a doubt, they play an essential part in our lives. We're better, happier people as a result of our friendships, but can it be possible that we're healthier, too?

The answer is a resounding yes. Studies have linked strong social connectedness with positive measures in areas as varied as motor skill retention, cancer survival, general immune function, memory preservation, and overall longevity.[4] That a healthy social life holds sway over our physical and mental wellbeing should come as no big surprise. We are social animals, after all.

So what happens to us then when we detach ourselves socially? To be sure, modern life encourages us to be antisocial. Individual homes and garages ensure that we need not meet our neighbors. Online ordering permits us to avoid public shopping. Television and streaming Internet mean we can conveniently enjoy entertainment in the seclusion of our own homes. Add to this picture the fact that we're increasingly a nation of movers and uprooters, finding ourselves far from the families and social networks of our youth.

As for the science, research shows that isolation has been linked to higher risk for Alzheimer's disease and heart disease.[5] One ambitious meta-analysis of 148 studies[6] showed a relationship between isolation and a higher risk of mortality. In one of those studies, researchers surveyed 4,775 adults in Alameda County, near San Francisco.[7] The subjects completed a survey that asked about social ties such as marriage, contacts with extended family and friends, and group affiliation. Each individual's answers were translated into a number on a "social network index," with a high number meaning the person had many regular and

ENVISIONING YOUR FIRE CIRCLE

Who would you include in your fire circle? What are the activities, values, stories, and rituals you're centered around or would like to cultivate? How would you describe the energy that pervades your community of friends? What about these relationships are enriching and sustaining for you? What do you offer to those in your circle?

close social contacts, and a low number representing relative social isolation. The researchers then tracked the health of the subjects over the next nine years.

Since the participants had varying backgrounds, the scientists employed mathematical techniques to isolate the effects of risk factors such as smoking, socioeconomic status, and reported levels of life satisfaction. The results were striking. Over the nine-year period, those who placed low on the social network index were twice as likely to die as individuals who had placed high on the index, but had otherwise similar risk factors. The researchers found that low social connectedness appears to carry the same increased risk as smoking and alcohol consumption.

Even group exercise appears to offer a significant boost in endorphin production over solitary exercise. In a study of rowers at Oxford University, those who performed rowing exercises in a group showed double the pain threshold than the solo rowers. The researchers attribute the extra endorphin rush to the social bonding, similar to that found in other collective physical endeavors, like hunting and dancing.

Our basic sleep quality is also influenced by strong social connections. In one study, those who described themselves as lonely experienced "increased nighttime vigilance."[8] There's plenty of evolutionary sense to explain this link between sleeping well and feeling secure in our social environment. Without the protection of a group, sound sleep must have been much more elusive.

The truth is, we need each other. As the adage goes, there's power—and evidently good health—in numbers. But is it possible to have too much of a good thing?

DUNBAR'S NUMBER

Primatologists have often noted that nonhuman primates live in small, tight-knit social groups of varying sizes. It's an extraordinary fact that the number of members within a group is not random but dependent on the size of a primate's prefrontal cortex. That is to say, the larger a primate's frontal lobe, the more social interactions the primate can manage.[9]

In 1992, British anthropologist Robin Dunbar figured the same principle ought to apply to human primates as well. Using the predictive value of neocortex size, he came up with a maximum "mean group size" of one hundred fifty and an "intimate circle size" of twelve.[10] Hypothesis in hand, he then compared his prediction with anthropological literature and reports from current-day hunter-gatherer societies to best approximate the social behaviors of our Paleolithic ancestors.

For the most part, Dunbar's predictions held true. Turns out the upper limit for human social cohesiveness is groups of about one hundred fifty, a number that has been validated throughout history when grouping size was critical for survival. History provides several examples involving intense environmental or economic pressure—like war (Roman maniples contained around one hundred sixty men) or early agriculture (Neolithic farming villages ran about one hundred fifty deep).

While Dunbar's Number has received some widespread recognition in the mainstream media, a group of one hundred fifty still can be overwhelming for a social circle. As previously mentioned, the hunter-gatherer existence self-regulated on groups made up of twenty-five to fifty members. Too few members made hunting unfeasible (as fit as he was, Grok wasn't taking down a buffalo by himself, let alone lugging it back to camp), and foraging became more effective the more hands committed to the task. A hunter-gatherer group had to be mobile and lean, able to follow the game when it moved. It had to be socially cohesive; people had to coordinate hunts, forage outings, and divvy up food. A large, ranging, sloppy group would mean more weak links, and in a social framework where every member was integral to the success of the whole, it simply wouldn't work out. A hunter-gatherer group that grew too big would simply become two hunter-gatherer tribes rather than languish and fail.

SOCIAL DISTORTION

Overstepping our natural bounds is essentially what makes us human. But what about overstepping Dunbar's Number? Can it increase stress? We see it in farm animals, whose increasing group size past optimal levels increases damaging behavior such as feather pecking in hens and tail biting in pigs. Granted, we are neither chickens nor pigs, but we, like other animals, are still sensitive to our environments.

Agriculture no doubt pushed our social limits by forcing us into crowded villages, but it's only recently that our social networks have undergone another,

> ## The researchers found that low social connectedness appears to carry the same increased risk as smoking and alcohol consumption.

even more drastic shift in size and composition. We're reconnecting online with childhood friends from years ago. We're getting text messages from twenty different acquaintances on a single day. Are we equipped to handle this sort of thing? Are we negatively impacting the quality of our social interactions? Are we spreading ourselves too thin? Or do social media platforms like Facebook and Twitter allow us to transcend, or tinker with, previously immutable biological limitations? Perhaps.

I'm reminded of how working memory describes the temporary engagement of information for immediate cognitive tasks like learning, reasoning, and calculating. Although theories on capacity vary, most people are limited to retaining four to seven "chunks" of working data. A chunk might be a single digit, a single word, or even a concept, but a few people can use advanced encoding techniques to expand the scope of each chunk. For instance, most people are able to repeat a seven-digit telephone number. But with memory techniques, a person might retain up to seven sequences of four or five numbers. This allows a person to remember thirty-five numbers instead of seven. The neurological bandwidth hasn't increased—the brain hasn't physically grown larger—it just utilizes the available bandwidth with greater efficiency.

Maybe Facebook and other social media offer the chance to make greater use of the available "socializing chunks" in our brain. Those seven chunks of available bandwidth are always going to be there, but it's what you put inside that matters. Perhaps tools like Facebook allow us to "store" information on friends and family without taking up valuable mental real

YOU ARE HARDWIRED *for a supportive circle of family and close friends.*

MODERN DISCONNECT: *an abundance of potential friends, mates, lovers, acquaintances, and business partners.*

PRIMAL CONNECTION: *reassess your inner circle, and rid yourself of the energy drainers.*

estate. I don't think that's either good or bad. Shoot, the reason we developed the written word was to avoid having to remember minutiae.

But I contend that we still on some level adhere to the spirit of Dunbar's number. Sure, we are capable of following thousands of people. It's done every day on Facebook and Twitter and other social media platforms. But few, if any, of us possess the emotional wherewithal to be involved with more than perhaps fifty people in any meaningful way. Go ahead, jot down a list of your current relationships—the ones you can quantify as meaningful and reciprocative—and see how many you come up with. Your number will likely be in the single or double digits. A 2009 study for the *Economist* found that even Facebook users with five hundred or more friends typically only interacted (commented on or "liked" postings, etc.) with seventeen people (males) or twenty-six people (females); and in two-way direct communication, interacted with only ten friends (male) or sixteen friends (female).

Now you may say social media has its merits. I agree. We don't always have time to reach out to our friends individually. Sharing a bit of ourselves "en masse" makes people feel they know what's going on in your life (and vice versa). Sometimes staying connected informally with status updates and messages is enough to get through a busy time or to get the ball rolling after a long hiatus and spur a real get-together. If you have a far-flung group of loved ones, it's nice to have creative ways to stay in touch and in each other's lives. I can personally testify to the power of an online community with Mark's Daily Apple. It's gratifying

MEETING OF THE MINDS

Did you know those few minutes you spend chatting up a stranger is enough to synchronize your brain waves? Studies show that a speaker's MRI brain activity is spatially and temporally coupled with that of a listener when they communicate, a coupling that quickly vanishes when they stop talking.[13] Feeling even a vague sense of connection with a stranger has been observed to generate a physiological synchronization.

to see members meet in person at our annual PrimalCon weekends. But that's the thing: you need to balance cyber time with in-person time. Chatting online or through email differs wildly from face-to-face interaction. Everything is calm and measured. There's little room for incidentals, mistakes, or purposeful, reflective pauses. You lose the physical contact and the body language cues, potentially running the risk of distorted and disoriented communication. Simply put, emoticons just don't stack up to the real thing.

Other more serious problems arise when virtual relationships displace or disrupt actual, real-life relationships. A poll taken by *The New York Times* found that electronic media influenced one out of seven spouses to spend less time

> **Agriculture no doubt pushed our social limits by forcing us into crowded villages, but it's only recently that our social networks have undergone another, even more drastic shift in size and composition.**

with their partners, and one of ten parents to shortchange time with their kids.[11] What do we miss when we step away from dinner to check how many "likes" our last Facebook update received, take yet another phone call, or check email? What do we give up when family members retreat to their respective devices each night? What do we forgo when we spend a road trip immersed in a DVD player or an iPod? What impact is there when people can't stand in line, sit at the airport, or even walk the dog without staring at or talking into an electronic device?

There's more, actually, than the immediate missed opportunities, neglected obligations, and disappointed loved ones. We aren't only giving up what's in the moment, but also the capacity to later attend to people and events with the same mental energy and focus when we finally disengage ourselves from our technological distractions. After all, a taxed brain peters out more quickly. How much energy do we give to our gadgets, and how little is left for the real priorities in our lives?

The fact is, we're still the same social creatures our ancestors were, with the same hunger for visceral connection. Culture and innovation, in service of human wellbeing, are amazing forces. But their effects must be checked by our natural needs. Innovation should serve us and give us a better life. It's time to return to a more original gauge of social wellbeing. It's time to recalibrate our lives toward genuine connections. We can then foster the relationships that really matter and the primal conditions that help them thrive.

REASSESS AND RECALIBRATE

What we intuitively know, research indeed confirms: our "best" experiences in life are those we share with others.[12] It isn't the awards and accolades but the birth of our children, the day we met or married our partner, or the amazing friendship that has grown over the years. However, does our calendar and mental focus reflect this truism?

In recalibrating your priorities, it's important to look at where your time goes, but don't forget about your energy and focus as well. Is the weekend really family time if you are simultaneously worrying about work or texting for long stretches? Time matters, but you have to have your head and heart in the game if it's really going to count. In our multitasking culture, it can be a hard impulse to tame. Nonetheless, your relationships will be better for it.

Ultimately, giving our relationships complete attention means upping our game entirely. What would our relationships look like if we brought the full force of our creativity and humor, the whole range of our curiosity and adventure to them? What if we left work *at work* and limited technology use to certain hours of the evening and weekend? Have you been stuck in a rut too long to even imagine this? Your family and friends are infinitely more interesting and would love to have you back.

Start now by distributing your energy wisely. Invest in the people closest to you and the relationships that serve your wellbeing the most. It's so easy to spread ourselves thin these days. There's a sense we should be expanding our social networks exponentially every year to be successful. As many amazing people as there are in the world, it just isn't feasible. We'll have great encounters with any number of people in our lives, but we need to make a conscious choice about who (and what) is most deserving of our energy. If you have five hundred

Facebook friends but can't make it to your child's piano recital without updating your wall, it's time to reassess your priorities.

In Grok's time, there was a scarcity of human contact. There was limited potential for relationships, and hence experiences were more concentrated. Now we have the potential to "friend" thousands—every person you ever came in contact with, from the guy who sat behind you in third grade to your dry cleaner—not to mention the random stranger who for some reason wants to be your friend. It becomes yet another abundance-scarcity mismatch with our genetic expectations.

The challenge for the new hunter-gatherer in the Primal Connection (that's you!) is to identify those people with whom you resonate, with whom you have a connection, and to foster those relationships, and to be willing to de-emphasize extraneous relationships. We're talking about Habit #1, Take Responsibility, which includes the people you allow access into your life. That goes for virtual friends, real-world friends, and acquaintances alike. It becomes critical not only to your wellbeing but in some cases to your success to surround yourself with good people—people who are supportive, uplifting, and from whom you can learn and feel great about their contributions.

CONNECTING WITH THE PAST

Maybe you still use your grandmother's measuring spoons or your grandfather's worn tackle box. On the walls of your home, there might be photos of generations past. Perhaps you keep a few books, a painted plate, or a woodcarving that was handed down. Likewise, you may have practices that have become conscious or subconscious family ritual. Or cook an old family recipe during the holidays or organize your tools the way a parent or grandparent once did. Whatever the means, we're preserving a bit of our history. These valued relics and simple rituals connect us to deeply personal stories. They allow us to participate in a continuity of memory and affection that fills us individually and reaffirms the ancient and adaptive value of holding the past within the present.

For example, I had one friend who, over time, just did not resonate well with me. Little things that he would say in a lighthearted, joking manner often left me feeling violated—accused of something or scolded for doing something better than he could. (As the saying goes, many a truth is spoken in jest.)

When we finally had a climactic altercation, I realized the energy differences between us and could no longer justify our friendship. I had to sever the ties. In doing so, I realized then that not only is it appropriate to surround ourselves

> " Ultimately, giving our relationships complete attention means upping our game entirely. "

with people who are supportive, upbeat, and positive, it's also appropriate to release those people who bring you down.

You don't have to have a finite, tangible, identifiable reason. In some cases it can be just a feeling (Habit #6, Trust your gut). The relationship may have just run its course and that's it. Or it might be that you no longer feel that you are getting from the relationship what you should be getting. Of course, there is give and take in any relationship, but when the giving greatly outweighs the receiving, you know there's a problem. So, to reiterate, it isn't just a matter of surrounding yourself with good people, but also recognizing who represents dead weight, the ones who drag on your happiness, your success, your wellbeing, and your health. You may know them as drama kings and queens, the energy drainers, the crazy makers, those who take, take, take, and never give back. Bottom line: love and friendship should be energizing, not draining.

Your challenge is to identify the top dozen or so people in your life whom you love and want to keep near and dear to you, and upon whom you would gladly lavish the majority of your social time and energy. These are the people for whom you would do just about anything—your spouse and children, for instance. They are the people you would want surrounding you on your deathbed. This is serious stuff—let's call it your inner circle. There is no obligation to include family members in this group "just because" they are blood. If you don't like them and wouldn't choose them otherwise, don't include them. Likewise, you may want to include certain close friends. These are the people you are happy for when they succeed, you will stick with during times of failure, and with whom you feel comfortable listening to and to whom you may speak your mind freely. These are the people who respond

IS OBESITY CONTAGIOUS?

It isn't necessarily the news we want to hear, but it makes intuitive sense. Several studies in the last decade have shown our social circle can significantly impact our weight.[14] The heavier our friends and family, the more likely we are to gain weight and remain heavy. On the flip side, the thinner our friends are, the more likely we are to be thin or be successful in our efforts to lose weight. Research into group weight loss (e.g., "team" competitions for workplace health programs) reveals weight loss tends to cluster.[15] In other words, we tend to feed off the success (or foundering) of those around us.

What can you do if those around you don't value physical health? It's important to dial in your expectations of others. Asking friends and family to support you in your goals on the one hand can set both of you up for failure. It's unfair and unreasonable to rely on someone else for our motivation. If they offer their genuine support and even use your example to inspire themselves toward healthier living, that's great. If not, it doesn't suggest the end of your relationship. Above all, you're responsible for your own choices.

Find people to add to your social circle who are on a similar journey, who can offer the perspective and support your existing network can't. Not every person in your life needs to share in this journey. Nonetheless, the powerful message in these studies suggests we can be a catalyst for change in others. Maybe they won't be in lockstep with us throughout the process, but our efforts can motivate others to think differently about their health potential and lifestyle choices. Even if it's months or years until they act on this new frame of reference, you've helped plant a seed for their wellbeing by honoring your own commitment to health.

in kind to you, and who you know you can truly depend upon should the going get tough.

After establishing your inner circle, consider the people you would like to place in your social circle. This circle will number a maximum of two dozen and will consist of those with whom you would like to nurture a meaningful, reciprocative relationship. These are the people with whom you might invite to a movie, hike a trail, or go out to dinner and enjoy some conversation.

Outside of your strong friendships, it feels great to build relationships with the people and places you do business with, too. There's something to be said for having a good rapport with your plumber. Likewise, it's helpful to have a doctor who's seen you through the stages and changes of your life. Sometimes we are so focused on finding a bargain that we often cheat ourselves out of better, more personal service. Ditto for buying locally. It might cost a bit more than the big-box offerings, but the convenience, the sense of connection, the personal service, and the support of your local economy counts for a great deal too.

Get to know your neighbors and coworkers. You'd think it's a given, but I increasingly find it's a stretch in our culture. We're absorbed in our own responsibilities. We're new to the job or area. We don't want to seem pushy. That nosy neighbor lady you try to avoid might be mildly annoying for surface encounters, but she's also the one who would go out of her way to keep an eye on your house or watch out for your kids. Injecting some authentic social enjoyment into work relationships can have a profound effect on not only team productivity, but also overall job satisfaction.

And, finally, the optimal size of your social circle is not an absolute number, but an estimate. We each operate with a different barometer when it comes to personal happiness and fulfillment. Some people thrive just fine in smaller social circles and experiences. They are often the same people who adapt better to increasing social isolation as they age. You'll know you're in the right ballpark if your social life promotes creativity, efficient collaboration, reciprocation, and happiness.

Love is exactly as strong as life.

JOSEPH CAMPBELL

FILLING THE SOCIAL WELLBEING

WE KNOW THE TIME WE spend with people matters. We can give them our full presence. We can infuse our relationships with more affection and creativity. But filling in the calendar and practicing our emotional focus seems to take us only so far. What else goes into building a strong fire-circle community? What else can ground us in a solid sense of connectedness? How else can we absorb the lessons of elders in our group and pass on our stories and rituals that shape our identity?

For our ancient ancestors, ritual was the key to social cohesion. It imposed an agreed upon order to life. It established common ground and constructed a group identity. Today, celebratory customs preserve the elements of family and community strained by such modern realities as long work hours and long distances between family members. Let's explore the possibilities, starting with seizing the moment.

Our hunter-gatherer ancestors (as well as traditional societies today) lived in a culture of immediacy, meaning life was lived around what could be found and created in the moment. Food was foraged instead of stored. Structures were erected as temporary shelters in keeping with periodic migration. Relationships, too, were continually recreated and reaffirmed through day-today contribution and interaction. Kinship was an ever-evolving relationship, not a fixed status.

What would it look like if we applied this "immediacy" to our close relationships today? What if we saw every day as a chance to remake our relationships in the present moment? So often we allow the responsibilities and routine of life to throw us into autopilot. It's important, now and then, to find a way to break the script of everyday life and refocus our relationships. Maybe it means time alone with a spouse, best friend, or individual child. Alternatively, we might recharge a connection best by seeing the relationship against a different backdrop—a couples' weekend, a team sport, or a family vacation. To follow, a few more fun suggestions on how to reconnect.

WAYS TO RECONNECT

Fill a family calendar—of nothing but fun. (The same idea works for couples and friendships.) Call a family meeting, hand out drinks with umbrellas, and fill in the dates—actual appointments—with everyone's favorite ideas. Whether it's a stay-cation week or a regular weekend, you won't regret the investment in your loved ones and their passions.

Use social media as a means to a more ambitious end. It's all in the strategy, balance, and follow-up. Try using social media to bolster relationships that already exist in your social circle. Use it to share the day-to-day funny stuff you'd forget to pass along in a conversation. And be selective about who you "friend."

Go old school. As inundated as we are with texts, emails, and social media, how about surprising someone with a bonafide piece of genuine mail—a postcard, a letter, a picture colored by your child, a greeting card, or care package. Think of it this way: "friends" send Facebook messages, but real friends shell out for the stamp.

Show up for live entertainment. In our ancestors' day, all entertainment was live. In fact, the whole point had more to do with the communal experience than the performance itself. Armed with the likes of OnDemand, Netflix, and iTunes, we moderns tend to forget this aspect of our humanity. It's so easy to get stuck at home in our insular bubbles, but we're missing out on whole dimensions of appreciation if we sit on the couch staring mindlessly at a screen. There's something uniquely satisfying about enjoying a play in the theater, a game in the arena, or a concert at the hall with others who enjoy the same pastime.

Look at it this way: strangers or not, we're all participating in a deeply ancient rite together. Getting up from our seats at the end, somehow we're connected to everyone in the audience who just had the same experience. That sensation is part of our human story. Better yet, make some live entertainment yourself. Host a game night. Ask a friend's daughter to play piano at your next neighborhood party. Organize a talent show at the next family reunion or otherwise chaotic holiday get-together. It will likely be memorable (and potentially hilarious).

Put yourself out there. Call it killing several birds with one stone. We stay shacked up in our homes, away from sun and scenery. How about giving the front porch some company? No front porch? How about lawn chairs on the driveway? Play with the kids in the front yard. Have your coffee or eat dinner out on the lawn. Use your condo community pool and grounds. Go for a stroll around the neighborhood. Stop. Talk. Catch up.

Keep the social hour social. Forget the need for a special occasion, novel recipes, and clever drinks. Have people over tonight and serve the same thing you'd serve yourself. Treat people more like welcome family than honored guests. (Trust me, they'll be more comfortable, too.) Be casual. Be spontaneous. My wife and I often share good times with another couple. They're the best dinner-party hosts you can imagine, routinely getting us involved with small chopping, grating, or other preparatory jobs soon after our arrival. The result is a casual, convivial ambiance in the kitchen that makes for a great party.

YOU ARE HARDWIRED *for immediacy and spontaneity.*

MODERN DISCONNECT: *the routine of life puts us on autopilot.*

PRIMAL CONNECTION: *change the backdrop and shake things up a bit.*

Build a fire. Life is just better with fire. We all know it. I'd venture to say a fire circle bears some kind of evolutionary imprint on our genes. We all gravitate toward it with no conscious will but a powerful instinct. A fireplace, a fire pit, a campfire, a bonfire, even candles in a pinch—they all do the same job. Take the fire circle to heart and invite a few old or new friends to spend a relaxing evening. I've noticed people tend to relax and open up by a fire in a way they wouldn't necessarily do in the broad lamplight. People share a little more, laugh a bit harder, and linger a lot longer.

MAKING NEW MEMORIES AND VALUING THE OLD

How many times do we take a pass on social opportunities—a blow-out vacation, a weekend outing, or even a spontaneous night out with friends? It sounds like fun. Often, we know it would be incredible, in fact. Money isn't even the issue most of the time. The problem? We just can't get over the hassle factor. When a friend invites the whole family to his cabin for a week, we imagine the seven hours it would take to pack for three kids. When a friend calls last minute with an extra ticket to the ball game, we think about the traffic and the stress of leaving work early instead of a chance to bond over live entertainment.

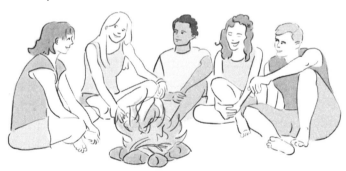

In balancing the pros and cons, however, we might not be giving the value of the experience its full due. Memories are, in fact, "durable goods."[16] They serve our wellbeing long after we've gotten caught up on laundry. The best measure of an adventure, researchers say, might even be found in the recollecting rather than the actual doing.[17] For example, a nightmare vacation makes for years of awesome stories and the affirmation of joint survival. In an age focused on convenience, we need to remember that life is about our experiences, however difficult or easy they may prove.

Likewise, remembering the traditions and meaningful times we've spent with our loved ones, in particular, can fill our emotional well. Research shows that wistful reminiscence boosts our self-confidence and enhances our feelings of connection.[18] Ritualizing our memories also provides a sense of continuity and meaning to our lives by encouraging us to see the past in a positive light.

Our hunter-gatherer ancestors continually reaffirmed the kinship ties they had to one another by contributing to the life of the band but also by celebrating the stories and the history of their connections to one another. Memories solidified and supported the group's identity. They also helped allow new members to integrate into the band. The same holds true today. Whether it's telling old stories around the dinner table or observing long-lived family and cultural customs, this emotional cohesion has the power to anchor our sense of self as well as strengthen familial and social connections.

We should acknowledge the value of memories, and—in light of the research—even ask ourselves periodically, "How am I doing on my memory investments these days?" The fact is, our recollections are more than fodder for good conversations or photo albums. They're emotional stores to get us through when times are tough or relationships are strained. Our memories are key supports to the resilience of our relationships and our own wellbeing.

THE BENEFITS OF BENEVOLENCE

Acts of generosity, research shows, don't just lead to emotional satisfaction; they actually promote physical health and healing. It's more than good karma, of course. There's evolutionary rationale to the warm fuzzies we get when we exercise our altruistic muscle. It behooved our ancestors to get along well and exhibit cooperation within their tribal groups. Even as the scale of social community expanded over time, a confluence of cultural motivation and genetic incentive appear to have still have favored "pro-social" behaviors. We're designed to be socially conscious and collaborative creatures.

Volunteering and other generous acts won't cure a disease, but they can help people with serious conditions cope with physical pain and ease their symptoms.[19] Other research links volunteering with higher levels of the immunity-boosting antibody immunoglobulin A (IgA) as well as decreases in blood pressure, stomach acid, and cholesterol counts. Researchers have long observed the emotional advantages of a generous disposition. The so-called "helper's high" is rooted in the release of endorphins. In keeping with this effect, those who volunteer report fewer stress symptoms and lower rates of insomnia.[20] Amazingly, even witnessing acts of charity has been shown to influence immune response—a phenomenon labeled the "Mother Teresa effect." Study participants who watched scenes of Mother Teresa helping others showed an increase in salivary IgA.[21]

Finally, it should be said that giving shouldn't be about obligation or necessarily about material exchange. Sulky obligation doesn't exactly inspire health and happiness in the giver—or gratitude and wellbeing in the recipient. Although studies in altruism have focused on volunteerism, generous acts can also be as small and personal as making your partner's favorite meal, holding the door for a stranger, or offering encouraging words to someone going through difficult times.

The idea here, we sense, is less about any particular action than it is about mindset. When it comes to benevolence benefit, it's truly the thought that counts. Adopting a magnanimous attitude can lift us out of the limited, and ultimately lonely individualism that can feel like, and truly be, a burden. As one study report highlights, common themes in volunteers' feedback include the satisfaction of making a connection and living with a sense of purpose.

Fostering genuine health involves more than pampering ourselves or checking off suggested acts for personal wellbeing. The act of giving places our potential for happiness outside of the restricted confines of our own lives. It extends our capacity for fulfillment and joy, beyond the daily details of our lives, to the good we can see and do in all that's around us.[22]

SECTION SUMMARY

The Inner Circle: The fire circle was the emblematic center of social life for our Paleolithic ancestors. The clan was typically made up of twenty-five to fifty members who engaged with neighboring groups for the resultant exchange of information about food, water, shelter, and danger. The cultural life and cosmology of the people was shared as participation was encouraged and rewarded within this social framework. Today, we are in jeopardy of depriving ourselves of the genuine nourishment of our social needs, through the very ease and extent of the virtual network. When we leave the dinner table (or—the horror!—not even sit down together to eat at all) to take that phone call, or check email, or invest hours in a video game or mindless TV, we are short-changing our closest and most important societal ties and emotionally starving ourselves in the bargain. Does our mental effort, our daily use of time, reflect the best of our experiences in life? Or are we giving it away to wider acquaintances and relative strangers? It's time to recalibrate our lives toward genuine connection.

Filling the Social Wellbeing: For our ancient ancestors, ritual was the key to social cohesion. Today, the ritual of telling family stories and recollecting memories fills our emotional storehouse with affection, meaning, and continuity that gets us through hard times and strained relationships. Our hunter-gatherer ancestors (and those of traditional societies today) also lived in a culture of immediacy, meaning life was lived around what could be found and created in the moment. What if we thought like a hunter-gatherer and saw every day as a chance to remake our relationship in the present moment? What if we reintroduced spontaneity back into our lives? What would you do with your leisure time? Maybe get away for the weekend with your partner, play with the kids on the lawn, or be part of the audience energy and go to a game, a concert, or a play? Don't allow the "hassle factor" to prevent you from making new memories. And invoke the ancestral heritage of warmth, relaxation, and the mystery of fire with a fireplace, a fire pit, a campfire, even candles. You'll feel better for it!

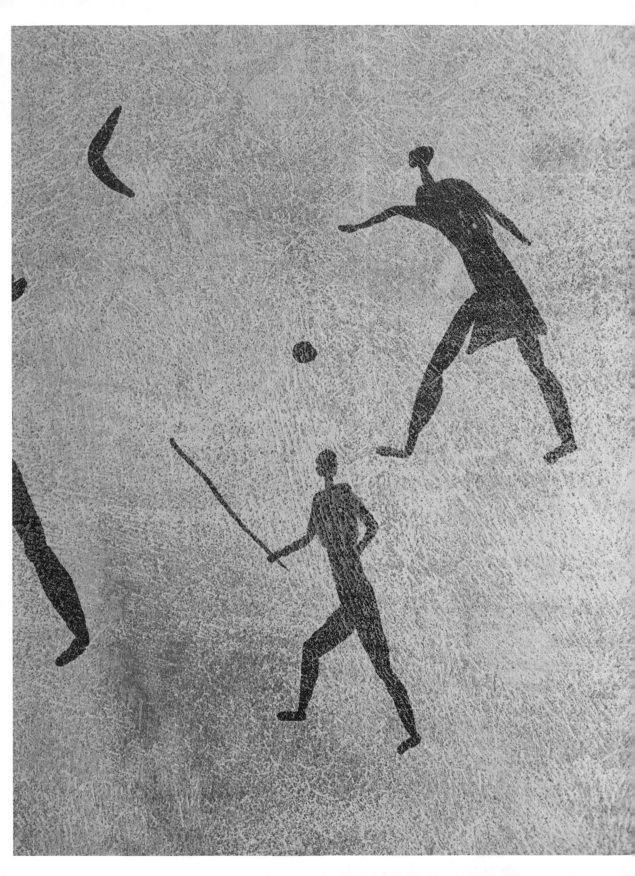

THE PLAY
CONNECTION

PLAY NURTURES OUR CREATIVE ENERGIES and strengthens our problem-solving skills. For tens of thousands of years, it was a vital component of communal living and social cohesion among our hunter-gatherer ancestors. Once the kill had been made, or the day's supply of roots, shoots, nuts, and leaves had been gathered, Grok played. The children might scamper around and chase each other. Adults might wrestle, race, have throwing contests, or even just lounge around and groom each other. This was pure, unadulterated leisure time, and there was plenty of it. However, our sense of play today is often considered a luxury or, even worse, "kids' stuff." You know there's a serious problem brewing when even your kids can't play without first checking their schedules. It's time to reclaim our birthright and play again.

Play is the highest form of research.

ALBERT EINSTEIN

PRIMAL PLAY

WE PLAY MORE THAN ANY other species, and we are one of the few that does not cease to play once we reach adulthood. Or at least that is what our genes expect. At first blush, it appears frivolous—fun for its own sake. But upon closer inspection, we learn that play has served as an innate survival skill throughout our evolution. We don't have fangs or claws or a hard shell—only our wits to help us maneuver through dicey situations. Play levels the field by providing an opportunity to experiment and process a variety of what-if scenarios. It helps us to test our limits and provides a wiring opportunity for the brain to plot strategies and escape routes. It also helps us blow off steam and reduce stress. We need play like we need sleep. Yet, like sleep, many of us deprive ourselves of it.

Indeed, play is an important part of the epigenetic influence on our genes in creating a lean, fit, happy, healthy, productive human body. But what is it exactly? By definition it is purposeless, all-consuming, and, most important, it's fun. This is the definition psychiatrist Stuart Brown gives in his book *Play: How It Shapes the Brain, Opens the Imagination, and Invigorates the Soul.* Brown is one of the few experts who have focused on studying the role of lifelong play. Over his career, he has studied how it has figured into a host of cultures and histories, and has compared the amusement patterns of various species. He calls play a "profound biological process" and presents evidence that play, across the span of our lifetime, literally designs our brains—forming new connections, creating new circuits, and organizing existing connections.

We know a deficiency of play can have dire consequences. Brown has done a lot of work in this area and compiled thousands of what he calls "play histories" on people. His studies reveal that children who were severely deprived of play demonstrated multiple dysfunctional symptoms, including lack of curiosity

> " Play levels the field by providing an opportunity to experiment and process different what-if scenarios. "

and social competency as well as uncontrollable emotions. What's more, Brown asserts that people who stopped playing in adulthood demonstrated a narrowing in their social, emotional, and cognitive intelligence. Conversely, highly creative and successful people lead lives filled with play.

In 2011, *The Wall Street Journal* ran a story that supports Brown's concept of play among successful individuals.[1] A number of up-and-coming CEOs from companies such as Google and Amazon attended play-focused Montessori schools in their early years, from preschool through first grade.[2] The difference in the educational method came down to what one CEO called "the joy of discovery" that instilled an interest in exploring, experimenting, and letting the imagination run wild.

We see this in the evolved workplaces of Silicon Valley—from whence some of the world's most innovative technology emanates. Beyond the stereotype of Ping-Pong tables, lava lamps, ropes course retreats, and casual dress codes, innovative companies like Google encourage a free-spirited, playful atmosphere. The company's technical employees are allocated one day a week to pursue creative projects unrelated to their core responsibilities. Not coincidentally, playing on the company clock has resulted in the

YOU ARE HARDWIRED *to play and learn throughout life.*

MODERN DISCONNECT: *a perception that play is just for kids.*

PRIMAL CONNECTION: *play, and play often.*

development of some of Google's most successful products, including Gmail and Google News.

Through play, we develop behavioral, intellectual, and emotional creativity and flexibility. Recall the discussion from Chapter 1 about the origination of the "cognitively fluid mind" sixty thousand years ago, which allowed us to invent culture and populate the globe. We've discussed at length how the pressures of adapting for survival shaped our genetic requirements for diet and exercise, but we cannot discount the contributions to progress that playtime has afforded. Play was and is the portal to refine our cognitively fluid minds, for it requires mental modeling, critical thinking, and creative innovation.

Children use play to experiment with the variety of feelings, experiences, and ideas they encounter in their development. We tend to discourage roughhousing and monkeying around, but these behaviors are important for children so they can learn boundaries and coping mechanisms. In the laboratory of play, they can even experience painful emotions and learn empathy, helping them to grow into more resilient adults. Experts use play therapy to help children

> **By definition play is purposeless, all consuming, and, most important, it's fun.**

process trauma, transition, and other difficult events. Research even shows that the physical manifestations of play help kids calibrate their appetite set point, protecting against childhood obesity.[3] And parent-child playtime delivers feel-good hormones to both parties, and enhances a child's sense of bonding and intimacy.

Though play has a long-term purpose, in the short term it has no particular point. That is to say, when you play—truly play—you have no attachment to the outcome. Notice young children who are just starting out in a team sport. They are learning the skill sets, and they're starting to move the ball around a little bit and starting to understand the concept of the game. They exhibit no attachment to the outcome. You might see the defense out in the field goofing around, maybe chasing butterflies. That's play. That's imagination and curiosity,

> ## "When you play—truly play—you have no attachment to the outcome."

that's being in the moment. Children commit 100 percent to their imagination and the fantastical roles inhabited in them. They enjoy it because they create it—and *feel* it—as real.

Left to their own devices, children exhibit an immense capacity for creative play, even with something as mundane as a cardboard box. It becomes an imaginary house, a fort, a ship. They can take something as simple as a mud puddle and turn it into an ocean, a lake, a crocodile-infested moat to the castle. Whatever it is, children exert a natural tendency to be creative and make something out of anything and amuse themselves freely for hours, simply for the sake of fun and exercising Habit #4, being in the moment. But once we see play becoming overly supervised and regimented, it becomes something else.

Consider the overly zealous high school soccer coach who steps in to coach a team and sees the raw talent and wants to mold and shape the players into champions. As the activity becomes more and more about winning (attaching an expectation to the outcome), the sense of play moves away. The game becomes more regimented and we soon see roster cuts, overtraining, burnout, and hurt feelings. The lesson here is we need to nurture our kids and encourage them to maintain their playful, youthful exuberance. And we need to maintain it in ourselves, too.

As we have learned, neglecting the play impulse doesn't bode well for us. Without play, Brown suggests, we become creatively rigid. We continually narrow the terrain of our cognitive musings, our social interactions, and physical life. The choice has inevitable consequences for our emotional wellbeing, our practical resilience, and our creative potential. In exalting the discipline of labor, we ignore how our original (and continuing) cognitive growth comes from play. Play isn't a distraction. It's the source of our personal and cerebral development— our potential for growth throughout life.

In adults, playfulness enhances intimate relationships by encouraging humor, lightheartedness, vulnerability, imagination, and ultimately a sense of connection.

You may recall a romantic relationship that fizzled due to nuance rather than major, tangible rifts. Even with ample time, attention, material contributions, healthy communication, and respect, relationship magic can easily vanish when play—and the laughter and free-spirited perspective it brings—is compromised.

I think that's the heart of what we lose as adults: the freedom of play, the pure release of it. We can coax ourselves to go play Frisbee in the backyard, get roped into dressing our kids' dolls for their latest tea party soiree, or even make ourselves join a summer baseball league or pottery class. In these cases, it isn't the action but the spirit that's lacking. Most of the time we're likely just faking it for the sake of the kids or our own sense of "healthy" obligation. (Obligation to play … how depressing is that?) We can be conscientious and simultaneously miss the point—and benefit—entirely.

YOU GOTTA BE KIDDING, MARK! I HAVE A 40-HOUR WORK WEEK AND A LONG COMMUTE!

It's dark when you leave for work, and it's dark when you get home. You say playing sounds all well and good, but you can't seem to figure out how to actually fit it into your busy life. As we build our careers and earn paychecks, many of us are asked to do things that are counterintuitive, that go against our hunter-gatherer genes that expect space, latitude, movement, and play.

As with any other life essential, we need to carve out the time to move our bodies, to get out of our linear brains, off of that spreadsheet and on to a much more expansive and open-minded approach to life. Play offers us an opportunity to do that. Do you have a weekend, an evening, a single hour? Can you multitask the Grok way, and include other members of your family so that you are playing, building your tribe, and creating quality time and memories all at the same time? If your schedule is so jam-packed that you can't even fit in an hour a week for play, you are probably taking on too many things and not practicing enough of Habit #2: Be selfish.

When we embrace play, we claim a better quality of life for ourselves. We decrease stress. We connect better with those around us. We get out more and get more out of what we do. We find more fun and meaning in our lives. And, later in life, it can even ward off cognitive decline and neurodegenerative conditions like Alzheimer's.[5]

Reclaiming play can at first seem intense and challenging, particularly if the muscle of your imagination has gone unused for a long time. We have more layers of stress, rationalism, and distraction to peel back than children, who can migrate effortlessly back and forth between the imaginative and the real, the instinctual and the rational—their connections between these worlds being more translucent and dynamic. We need to make that portal more accessible and clear out the mental space between concrete "reality" and fluid, open-ended play. Like a path in the woods, the more we travel it the more navigable it becomes, and the more instinctual our experience of it is. Play and humor gradually infiltrate life in a free-flowing way again. We rediscover our own orientation toward play—whatever form it most naturally and enjoyably takes in our personalities and circumstances.

NO ATTACHMENT TO THE OUTCOME

The idea of having no attachment to an outcome is a difficult concept for a lot of folks to grasp. And yet it becomes an important life strategy. When you look at studies done on centenarians that compare lifestyles, behaviors, and all other data points, you don't really find a lot of correlation among the diets or exercise patterns. Hey, some don't even exercise much, and others partake in a daily cocktail or smoked cigars. But the one thing that centenarians all seem to have in common is an ability to roll with the punches and overcome adversity.[6] It appears that this life skill to be able to move on after the loss of a loved one, a divorce, or the loss of a job is a particularly important strategy for living a long, happy, healthy, productive life. It's about going with the flow, it's about simply releasing attachment to the outcome. That doesn't mean you don't play hard. It doesn't mean that you don't get into a game and say, "I want to win this game." But it's the idea that after it's over, you move on with your life. No regrets. No ruing it. You simply move on.

Imagination will often carry us to worlds that
never were. But without it we go nowhere.

CARL SAGAN

THE PLAY OF ART

THE CREATIVE ARTS AS WE know them today likely stemmed from the early impulse to tinker. The purely pragmatic eventually made room for the artistic. Although we tend to think of our pre-Neolithic ancestors as living a life stuck in the dirt with no sense of refinement, we're far off course in that assumption. Artistry is indeed an anthropological indicator of modern behavior, but evidence of these inclinations date back tens of thousands of years before the Agricultural Revolution. As early as one hundred thousand years ago, our Paleolithic ancestors were creative, artistic, and inventive.[7] They painted caves and made jewelry from shells and bone fragments.

Wouldn't you know it, that natural impetus lingers to this day with practical—and sometimes dramatic—results for our physiological wellbeing. Far from being mere childish distraction, creativity and imagination are crucial to the development of advanced cognition, problem solving, and social empathy.[8] Imagination arms us through the tumult of adolescence, the disorientation of life's griefs, and all the ordinary dilemmas of everyday living. Yet, it also spurs us forward—toward higher goals and down more risky, but ultimately rewarding, paths. Its power allows the relief of momentary displacement and is a catalyst for long-term transition.

Such results suggest that fine-tuning our imaginative powers might reap more than relaxation benefits. What might be the cumulative effect of applying guided imagery and other imaginative practices to the body's functioning and balance? If we favor the path of prevention, then indulging, developing, and refining an active imagination might be a worthy Primal investment.

Specific instructions for an unstructured activity are impossible (and counterproductive), but there is a basic guideline: anything goes. Discover your own particular brand of play. Let it take many forms. For most of us, we'll naturally gravitate toward something we enjoy and excel at. If you tend to lean toward the cerebral, the next chapter on adrenaline pursuits is for you. But if you already push the envelope on outdoor pursuits, try finding pleasure in simply reading or painting. The point is, play is meant to add some balance to the predominant elements of your daily routine.

Let's start with your workday, where you probably spend the most time. When I talk about sharpening your spear (Habit #9), this isn't just about addressing your work ethic. It means your creative ethic as well. It means becoming a well-rounded person. Yet many of us have, by necessity in the modern economy, become specialists, concentrating our focus on a single star rather than the galaxy it occupies.

When it comes to the more mundane tasks, there is, indeed, hidden value in taking out the garbage, doing the dishes, chopping vegetables, fixing a loose board on your deck, even spending thirty minutes on the production line if you're the CEO. Pursue the highest expression of your talents by all means, but if your role is highly specialized, stressful, complex, or abstract, look around and see where you can pull back and then broaden your horizons.

One often doesn't apply the prevailing definition of play to growing a tomato, building a chair, or painting a fence. But anyone who has spent significant time creating with their hands—whether it be painting, carpentry, knitting, carving, or building—can appreciate the distinctive satisfaction it evokes. (Again, another hardwired response.) Picture our hunter-gatherer ancestors sewing clothes from animal sinew, forming vessels, or weaving baskets. They created paints and dyes. They chiseled spearheads

YOU ARE HARDWIRED *for artistic expression.*

MODERN DISCONNECT: *the daily grind leaves no time for self-expression.*

PRIMAL CONNECTION: *be in the now.*

from stone so brittle few of us can even imagine the deftness required. They meticulously whittled shafts to create efficient, aerodynamic spears. (Eat your heart out, Neanderthal!) They designed vast stretches of nuanced cave art.

As anthropologists suggest, human proclivities toward craft and artistry increased the odds of survival for individuals and their communities. A skilled spearmaker added obvious value. Yet those who could design jewelry or other adornment introduced "material metaphors" and "social technologies" that enhanced relationships and community identity as well as expanded the terms of inter-band negotiation.[9]

Bear in mind that handicraft, as wide a spectrum as it can encompass, isn't about routine chores or fix-its. There's a difference between grudgingly doing your own home repairs to save money and savoring the experience of meticulously renovating your master bathroom. It's about being a good steward, yes. It's also about the love of the craft. Artisans, hobbyists, and do-it-yourselfers are drawn to what they do on a subconscious level. They develop a reverence for the craft and even a relationship with the tools they use. Picking up a familiar tool feels comfortable, even calming. The balance of its weight in your hand feels sure. Sometimes the tools can become more personal than the items we build or create. The brush or needles, chisel or knife, spade or hammer become an unconscious extension of the self. The mind devises, but the hand itself thinks, designs, knows. In its fullness, we lose ourselves in the full physical experience of craft—in the sensory nuances, in the emotional associations, in the intuitive energy. I'd venture to say that we're the happier and healthier for these endeavors. It's in the craft that you find focus—or even flow.

A recent study conducted by the Center for Reducing Health Disparities at the University of California, Davis highlighted "the link between traditional artistic practices and mental and physical health."[10] Although examining such an association with the methods of standard research isn't a simple or clear-cut task, interviews suggested that traditional handicraft bears positive impact on measures like interconnected mind-

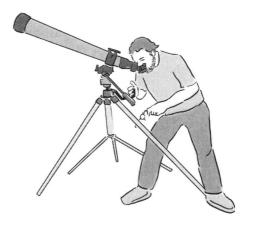

body awareness, spiritual and emotional growth, physical vigor, strengthening of personal and community identity, and therapeutic distraction from illness.

Of course, the fine arts—sculpting, painting, music, poetry—or cerebral pursuits such as reading and playing crossword puzzles, brainteasers, or chess all constitute play as well. As the saying goes, just do it.

THE CREATIVE PLAYGROUND

Use your imagination. Play, for all intents and purposes, is our continuing experiment in self-development. It gives us the opportunity to try on varying abilities, techniques, differences, even alternative lives—like children donning dress-up clothes. It paves the way for the rush and stretch of discovery—the revelations of our own possibilities, of the reality and depths of others, of the beautiful and confounding complexity of our world. Play finally brings us full circle, suggesting a life richly lived isn't a linear path but a spiraling journey that leads us forward and yet brings us time and again through familiar, ongoing patterns.

So, who do you want to be? Maybe a storyteller or a writer? A painter or a dancer? A master chef or a scientist? Your imagination allows all of these sorts of opportunities to develop and helps you zero in on what might be a special passion. Write a list of ten things that intrigue you, things you want to explore and know more about. Include dream jobs on your list. And include a couple of long shots. Astronaut? Go ahead, write it down. Now commit yourself to doing something an astronaut might do, even if it is just looking out over the night sky or perusing the science section at your local bookstore. In the process, you may discover another hidden passion. You want to be a writer? Join a poetry slam or enroll in a writers' workshop. Or maybe you enjoy food, and you're already a pretty good cook. Raise the bar and challenge yourself to whip up something new and different from a foreign land. Or create a new recipe, maybe several, take pictures of them, and put them all in your very own cookbook. Remember, this is play, which means there's no failure—only fun, and learning what works and what doesn't. It also means reduced levels of stress hormones and enhanced immune function, life satisfaction, and self-esteem.

Pick up a tool. Build a simple latticed shelter over your existing deck to eventually populate with vines or canvas; do some decorative tiling in your shower or bathroom counter; repaint your bedroom in some lively colors. As with art, home repair shouldn't be the private domain of licensed contractors. Pick up a tool and you lose yourself in its sensory nuances and intuitive energy. No wonder dinnertime comes and goes when you are in building mode! For more ideas, go to a big-box home-supply store and check out the ongoing series of free classes on assorted home improvement projects. YouTube videos are also great resources to give you sufficient guidance to do a simple project safely and successfully.

> " Far from being mere childish distraction, creativity and imagination is crucial to the development of advanced cognition, problem solving, and social empathy. "

Listen to music. Most of us have experienced the transformative effects of music. Whether a true evolutionary adaptation or a deeply embedded and heritable product of culture, music was—and remains—a profound contributor to our human story. Infants exhibit musical abilities that suggest a penchant for music is coded into our genes. The human voice was undoubtedly the first instrument, dating back at least sixty thousand years, while the oldest flute dates back thirty-five thousand years.[11] Evidence suggests that music strengthens social bonds through its role in ritual and celebration, and was likely involved in hunting, language acquisition, and even sexual selection for musical talent.[12] What's more, it moderates the stress hormones cortisol and epinephrine, lowers blood pressure and heart rate, and elevates growth hormone levels.[13] It's also proven to enhance the way you process language, verbal memory, and emotion.

Learn to play an instrument. Then there's the experience of making music yourself. According to Norman Weinberger, professor of neurobiology and behavior at University of California, Irvine, playing an instrument works several regions of the brain simultaneously and calls on a number of senses, including vision, hearing, touch, motor planning, emotion, and symbol interpretation.[14] According to Weinberger, this complex level of engagement could explain the ability of those with Alzheimer's who have retained the ability to create music when many other prominent memory functions are compromised.

Watch people. Head to a high-traffic public place such as an airport, train station, busy coffee shop, or high-rise office complex. Pack a lunch and enjoy the ever-changing scenery. What kind of game can you make of it? Guess their conversations? Their thoughts? Their occupations? Maybe even summarize their life stories?

Break for play. Can you bring a little of the Google workplace ethos into your work environment? Heed the recommendations to take regular cognitive breaks throughout the workday, and make them as playful as possible. Have ongoing, high-stakes challenges for excellence in Nerf basketball, turf putting, paper airplanes, freestyle rapping, one-legged stairwell ascending, or caricature doodling for display in the break room's Wall of Fame. If you have a lengthy commute, how about stopping off at that park playground once in a while? Take a spin through the jungle gym challenges, complete a par course, shoot a few baskets, or toss a few snowballs at your favorite targets before returning to the road.

Witness the wonder. Pay special attention when you expose someone—a child or an adult—to something awesome for the very first time. It could be acting as a tour guide for a visiting friend and seeing your hometown in a fresh, new way. Or taking a grandchild to a familiar place, made brand new again through their wonder. Or simply teaching a child to fly a kite or ride a wave. Absorbing that unmistakable look in a person's eyes, when they are filled with awe and satisfaction, can elicit a similar impact on you.

More ways to play. Take an art class, enroll in a comedy improv class, go to a play, spend the evening in a comedy club, read a book, solve a crossword puzzle, join a chess club. You get the idea. It's a big world out there. Go play!

Do one thing every day that scares you.

ELEANOR ROOSEVELT

PRIMAL THRILLS

HOW COULD LIFE FOR A hunter-gatherer be anything but an adventure? Just as our ancestors ventured to the edge once in a while, our genes expect the same from us. That's right, every once in a while, we need to do something that pushes our limits and expands our boundaries. The urge is as natural as it is stirring. I'm talking about an occasional adrenaline rush to refresh and reset your cognitive and emotional compasses. The sort that suspends you in the heady risk of action, where time seems to stop, or at least slows down considerably. I'm talking about the kind of thing where you are fully engaged in the moment and become raw awareness, where the heightening of the senses can feel like skating along a razor's edge that separates focus from fear.

There is indeed a certain thrill in testing our nerves, pondering how much farther down a darkening forest path we'll go until fear or practical thoughts win out. Extreme physical endeavors—like freestyle skiing, mountain biking, climbing, surfing, white-water rafting, and so on—do the same. Such activities depend on sensory acuteness. Obviously, I wouldn't recommend doing them without proper instruction, guided practice, and setting sensible limits. But in gaining mastery of these "sports," we feel out and fine-tune our perceptiveness. We learn to trust our gut, Habit #6. A matter of a couple degrees in one's lean on a steep hill can spell disaster for a skier. The angle and height of rifts in a white-water scene tell a kayaker how to navigate. A climber learns the subtle difference between the feel of a foothold that is steady and one that is compromised or too shallow.

In this way, extreme endeavors and other spontaneous, inspired physical activities take us out of the rational and plant us wholly in the sensory. As suggested by Diane Ackerman, noted naturalist and author of *Natural History of the Senses*, extreme athletes reference a sense of "cleansing" and "divestiture" when explaining what draws them to their passions. They enter that precipice between actual danger and exuberant experimentation, tempting fate to relish the thrill of the chase, holding back just enough that they can withdraw in time to save their skins.

So much of life these days is routinized, regimented, parceled out for maximum efficiency and order. We spend a lot of it on a comfortable, safe plateau: such is the opportunity modern life affords. Few of us face any real hazard in a day. Few of us experience shocks to the system, those fleeting moments of hormesis, and are confronted by our own mortality in material, appreciable ways, or with any regularity. For the most part, it's a profound benefit and historical boon to live in an age of unmatched certainty compared to that of our distant and not-so-distant ancestors. Yet, something in us feels the incongruity. We evolved facing threat. All those eons and thousands of generations molded our bodies and minds for acute risk and corresponding resilience. It's unnatural to live without it. Something in our genetic capacity languishes. Something in our inherent nature withers or, alternatively, rebels. We become bored, overtaken by a sense of detached fatigue and inexplicable ennui.

In response, we fabricate risk with meaningless social drama or do genuinely dangerous, irresponsible, and stupid things that offer nothing to our health or self-actualization. Or we quietly, unconsciously acquiesce. There's a price for this resignation, I think. As Ackerman puts it, "Where there is no risk, the emotional terrain is flat and unyielding, and, despite all its dimensions, valleys, pinnacles, and detours, life will seem to have none of its magnificent geography, only a length."[15]

In the end, risk, as irrational as it is, is intuitive. Without it, we live stuck, inert, fixed at center. We give up the chance to explore the wild peripheries of living—and the reinvigoration that adventure offers even when we come back to the base of everyday life. When you honor these impulses, you return to ordinary life refreshed and deeply appreciative of your secure surroundings, a warm shower, a nourishing meal, a group of friends to regale with your tales of adventure. We are indeed a species that thrives in dichotomy.

Risk doesn't have to be physical, of course, and I'm not suggesting you deliberately insert yourself in dangerous situations. I believe, however, that we benefit from activities that propel us to heightened mental and physical states, in which we further develop our often half-used senses and give ourselves over to a more primitive but powerful source of focus.

> **There is indeed a certain thrill in testing our nerves, pondering how much farther down a darkening forest path we'll go until fear or practical thoughts win out.**

Consider the sixteenth century's Portuguese explorer Ferdinand Magellan and his forty-three-thousand-mile journey to circumnavigate the globe. In search of a western route to the Spice Islands from Europe, he sailed down the South American coast—south, south, south into stormy seas and an increasingly brutal winter, with absolutely no idea where the southern tip was, or how long it would take to get there. Once around the continent, he fully expected to encounter the Spice Islands (near modern-day Indonesia) in short order, only to deal with an additional three months of sailing the endless (endless in the most profound sense of the word) waters of the Pacific.

Sitting here today, with Google Earth at our fingertips, it's almost impossible to comprehend such a mysterious, treacherous, perspective-altering journey. Closer to home, I can recall with great detail the looks on my kids' faces on the occasions of their first bike ride, first sleepover camp, and first time taking the car out solo. Certainly you have cherished memories of facing challenges, uncertainty, or even danger, and the resulting sense of personal accomplishment. Heck, I've failed numerous challenges, but grew from the experience of having tried.

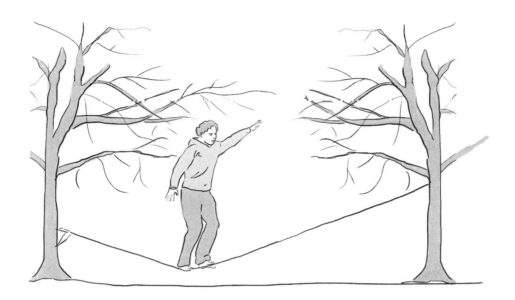

Like Magellan, we still possess our factory wiring for adventure—a continual desire to explore the limits of our physical and mental capabilities and our world in general.

What we are going for here is *calculated* risk. We access this through the physical realm because the intensity and graphic nature of physical challenges build confidence and bravery, virtues that can be applied to the other connections suggested in this book and life as a whole. Clearly, such risks are subjective, and you alone preside over your definition of what constitutes a calculated risk. A close friend of mine defines it as BASE jumping off El Capitan, Yosemite's nearly three-thousand-foot-tall granite monolith. We've hiked the trail to the top together, but I can't even bring myself to get close enough to the edge to watch his performance! Conversely, if you're the type to test the limits of your motorcycle skills by revving up to 120 mph on the interstate at midnight, you may need to question if you are distorting this primal urge for adventure.

Pushing the envelope demands that you access the flow state. To reiterate the disclaimer, there

YOU ARE HARDWIRED *to engage your fight-or-flight response with positive, intermittent stressors.*

MODERN DISCONNECT: *predictable, safe, comfortable modern life.*

PRIMAL CONNECTION: *pursue adrenaline-rush adventures!*

is no need to put your life in danger to access this state of mind. Psychology professor Mihaly Csikszentmihalyi asserts that your challenges must sync with your abilities. Something too easy will bore you, but something too difficult, too dangerous, and too far outside of your comfort zone will likely cause you to disengage and become consumed by fear or frustration.

I can sense very well where the limitations of my snowboarding abilities lie, and I always stay well clear of crossing that line into the danger zone. I accept the calculated risks of sliding down a mountain slope, do my very best to mitigate

> **Like Magellan, we still possess our factory wiring for adventure—a continual desire to explore the limits of our physical and mental capabilities and our world in general.**

these inherent risks by staying totally focused and cognizant of my limits. I believe strongly that the vast majority of "accidents"—not only in extreme sports but also in all physical activities—result from stupid mistakes rather than a natural consequence of the inherent risk. Often, the stupid mistake involved is the initial decision to attempt an endeavor with excessive risk. I respect and marvel at big-wave surfers, extreme skiers, and mountaineers, but I reject exceeding the limits of skill and common sense in the name of accomplishment.

A skydiving friend of mine related a serious accident where he sustained numerous broken bones and damaged organs but lived to tell about it. The cause was a malfunctioning parachute that opened only partially due to improper packing. He typically paid an attendant at the skydiving center twenty bucks to pack his chutes. He was saving time so he could take more jumps! Upon returning to the sport, he decided to assume that job himself.

Whatever your parameters are, it's essential to assess the risk-versus-reward factor carefully and harness all the concentration you can muster—not only to achieve the exalted flow, but to be safe. The goal is to proceed accordingly through exciting physical challenges, experience the thrill of being in the zone or the flow, increase your competency at your favorite activities, and broaden your horizons to pursue exciting new challenges in the future.

As you pursue Primal Thrills in the adrenaline-rush category, a certain element of physical risk and danger may be involved. But the same holds true anytime you zone out in daily life. In fact, when you access the flow state and test your boundaries, you invariably improve your ability to focus, heighten your awareness of risk and danger, and access an elevated mental and physical state where your attention becomes primal instead of scattered.

If you've walked by the pickup basketball game in the park every day at lunch but never summoned the guts to play, jump in there one time and see if you can hang. Hey, you might get embarrassed, but you can hold your head higher than that guy who walks by every day and never takes his shot. Did you high jump, throw the shot, or pole vault "back in the day"? See if you can reawaken old passions like these through a local community sports program.

If you already have a certain level of devotion to serious physical challenges, see if you can take things to the next level. In *Bone Games: Extreme Sports, Shamanism, Zen, and the Search for Transcendence,* author Rob Schultheis discusses how being pushed to the edge of his physical limits allowed him to access a higher level of consciousness and peak performance. He relates accessing the flow or the zone during a perilous mountain climbing experience. Having suffered significant injuries in a fall, he was stuck in the wilderness with a dangerous storm approaching. Inspired at a primal level by his dire circumstances, he proceeded to descend a treacherous mountain pass with uncanny speed and mastery. In Schultheis's words:

> Something happened on that descent, something I have tried to figure out ever since, so inexplicable and powerful it was. I found myself very simply doing impossible things: dozens, scores of them, as I climbed down Neva's lethal slopes. Shattered, in shock, I climbed with the impeccable sureness of a snow leopard, a mountain goat.

When Schultheis healed his body and returned to the scene of his adventure later, he could scarcely believe what he had accomplished and the danger level that he'd barely blinked at.

To follow are a few more suggestions for Primal Thrills, but I want to emphasize imagination and creativity on this connection. There are plenty of ways to push your boundaries in your everyday life, maybe volunteer to do some public speaking or ask for that much-deserved raise. But overall I want you to think about outdoor, natural settings, minimal logistics, and pursuing the purity of the experience. See if you can call up a healthy bit of fear, anxiety, and uncertainty of outcome—within reason of course—in order to access a higher level of consciousness and peak performance.

Amusement parks. Challenging the law of gravity is a surefire way to get a safe rush. Granted, the long lines and cotton candy stands might not be as badass as Schultheis scrambling down a dangerous slope during a lightning storm, or modern-day Magellans racing in the Vendée Globe. However, the waterslides, the roller coasters, and the ever-more sophisticated and gasp-inducing contraptions rising from your nearest amusement park are a harmless way to get crazy and extreme. What's more, your genes don't know the difference between a life-or-death adrenaline rush and a simulated one at the amusement park.

Night hike. Join a local recreation group that offers organized night hikes or snowshoe outings. Expect some sweaty palms, an elevated heart rate, and jittery nerves as you enter into the unfamiliar world of darkness. As you proceed with your adventure, a sense of focus and peace will edge out your initial fears. In a short while, your hardwired instinct and sensory acuity will take over and you'll realize you're somehow able to balance your body deftly along a dark, rocky trail. You'll hear every small sound and identify the exact source. As other long-buried, primal abilities present themselves, you'll gain courage and confidence that is hard to acquire via the quarterly sales contest or adult softball league playoffs.

Competition. Anything that gets your competitive juices going will facilitate a flow experience. Join that pickup basketball game, organize a neighborhood Ping-Pong tournament, or pull the trigger and enter a mud run, beach volleyball tournament, or mini triathlon.

Jump off something. Jumping from an elevated perch into water could be the quintessential Primal Thrill. Find a river, lake, or ocean with rocky shorelines and a suitable perch from which to launch. Failing these options, go for the high-diving board at a local swimming pool. Caution and good sense are advised here. First, if you haven't seen anyone else jump from the spot, you're taking a risk! Second, I go feet-first when jumping into any body of water besides a swimming pool. If the water is not crystal clear, I first dive down and thoroughly examine the landing area to ensure it's of a safe depth and there are no debris or protruding objects beneath the surface.

While it's hard to do damage jumping from 10 feet or less, anything over that height requires correct form to prevent injury. For example, even something as innocuous as hitting the surface with your arms outstretched can tear a rotator cuff when you are a couple stories high and beyond. Also, it's a great idea to wear Vibrams or sneakers to protect your bare feet from impact trauma.

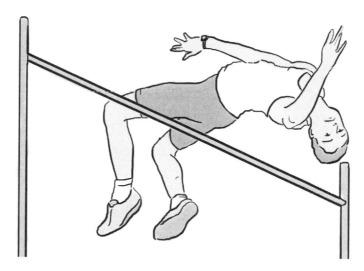

Martial arts. This affords mind/body benefits along with all-around physical conditioning. Breaking bricks—what a great metaphor for becoming a more powerful and confident person!

Mini adventure race. Choose three or more modes of transportation and establish a challenge to go from point A to point B using various forms of locomotion (human-powered only). For example, take a bike ride to the lake, swim to the opposite shore, hike the perimeter to return to your bike, and then ride back home. Throw in a skateboard, scooter, or—if you have winter conditions—snowshoes, cross-country skis, and ice skates. City-dwellers can try this: hike two blocks to a building with twenty-plus stories and accessible stairs.

EXPANDING YOUR COMFORT ZONE

Get an oversized piece of paper—an artist's sketch pad, butcher paper, whatever … it doesn't have to be fancy. Draw a large circle in the middle of the paper. Inside, title the circle "Comfort Zone." Write the names of fifteen skills that are currently inside your comfort zone—an arbitrary boundary that your mind has created, inside of which you feel safe, confident, relaxed, and risk-free. Can you run three miles comfortably? Rattle off twenty-five pushups? Program computer software? Sell real estate? Write screenplays? Write your particulars down in the circle if they are routine for you. Then, think about related endeavors that are outside your comfort zone that you wish to achieve—run six miles, do fifty pushups in one effort, or perhaps actually sell your screenplay. Write down these ideas outside of the circle.

That was the warm-up stuff; now go beyond fitness and professional skills into matters of personal conduct, career, and relationships. Have you been getting vibes from the guy at the coffee house, but hesitant to ask him out? Write it down outside the circle. Do you comfortably communicate with your teenager about intimate personal matters, or do you wish things could be more open on that front? Keep going with anything that comes to mind. Refer to the Primal Thrills suggestions, as well as the summaries of the previous sections of the book, and write down some important connections you would like to make that are outside your comfort zone. These don't all have to be quantifiable; you could write about being more patient, taking criticism better, or improving your listening skills. Don't worry, you don't have to display the completed worksheet on your front door; this is a private exercise to get you in touch with some personal growth opportunities.

Now, circle five of the most important things lying outside of your comfort zone that you would like to bring inside your comfort zone immediately. Have that difficult talk with your boss or loved one; achieve an ambitious fitness goal; approach the coffee clerk; and so forth. If necessary, write some notes next to the item with specifics on how you plan to take immediate action. As you tackle each of these challenges, realize that your comfort zone grows larger and larger. Essentially, this represents your lifelong goal—to tackle new challenges continually and to expand your comfort zone by doing so!

Climb and descend the staircase, then hike another two blocks to a new building and repeat.

Nature challenges. Mountain climbing, rock climbing, water sports (swimming, surfing, standup paddling, waterskiing, wakeboarding, wakesurfing), and winter sports (downhill and cross-country skiing, ice skating) all entail synchronizing your physical efforts with natural forces—going with the flow. You haven't lived until you have tried standup paddling or wake surfing (yep, sans rope behind a ski boat). Moving within a naturally varied environment like water virtually demands that you transition out of an analytical state into a flow-like state.

Photo scavenger hunt. A game director is required to administrate this game. Form several teams (the more, the better!) of two or three people. Arm each team with a digital camera. The game director prepares a list of items to photograph, with corresponding point values for degree of difficulty. On the photo list, describe points of interest in your area, riddles that reveal a specific location, and outrageous, difficult-to-orchestrate situations (for instance, a photo of a team member getting shampooed at a hair salon; eating watermelon with a stranger on a bus bench; sitting astride a Harley Davidson motorcycle; with a non-domesticated animal visible in the picture; or submerged in a pool holding a bag of potato chips).

Begin by distributing the photo lists to the teams, start the clock, and establish a return time of two to three hours. Upon return, each team's photos are evaluated, points tabulated, and a winner declared. Printing out the photos onto a collage for each team makes for a great souvenir!

Slacklining. It's such a simple endeavor, but one of powerful symbolism. A slackline is a flat nylon tightrope a couple inches wide that you suspend from two anchor points, such as trees, or strong posts or poles. As the name suggests, the line is not taut under the user's weight; rather it will stretch and recoil under the load. It looks easy, but it's a tremendous challenge to simply mount the line and keep your footing. The dynamic tension in the line can send you flying off with the slightest disturbance to your center of gravity.

Slacklining is an activity that engrosses you immediately. An approach that's too casual will send you flying off the rope; try too hard and you might soon find your legs doing the dreaded sewing machine (uncontrollable twitching). But when you can get into the sweet spot of balance and start taking steps up and down the line, it's a blissful, connected feeling. Search YouTube for "Slackline World Cup" and you'll see the amazing exploits of "trickliners" who use the line like a trampoline, launching to perform aerial tricks and then landing gracefully back on the skinny line.

Speed golf. Wait until twilight and tee off on an empty course. Carry a junior golf bag with just a handful of clubs. Jog from shot to shot and play quickly, but at the same time making your best effort to score well, including putting. Count one point for each stroke and each minute on the course to produce a total score. World champion Jay Larsen once shot a 71 on a regulation-length course in thirty-seven minutes, for a speed golf total of 108!

Ultimate Frisbee. If you haven't tried it, you are missing out on one of the most enjoyable games around! All ages and ability levels can play safely together, with minimal equipment or logistics, in groups of varied numbers. I recommend a minimum of six players and a maximum of sixteen. Depending on the size of the group, a field of 50 to 100 yards length and 35 to 50 yards width is ideal. The game (the proper term is simply "Ultimate," since Frisbee is actually a brand name) is somewhat like soccer with a flying disc. Teams try to score a goal by covering the length of the field passing the disc and crossing the end line.

You can pass forward or backward to any open teammate but cannot run if you are the passer. If a team on offense drops the disc, the other team takes possession on the spot immediately and tries to pass to open players and get across the opposite end line—it's nonstop action! Players should match up with opponents appropriately by size and ability, covering players from the opposing team in man-to-man defense style. However, no physical contact with an opponent is allowed except incidental contact going for the flying disc. These rules allow for the full and safe inclusion of a diverse group.

SECTION SUMMARY

Primal Play. We play more than any other species, and we are one of the few that does not cease to play once we reach adulthood. Play is and has always been vital for our survival and advancement as a species. It is part of our cognitive survival set, providing opportunities to learn, process what-if scenarios, experiment, and solve problems. But in the moment, true play has no particular purpose. When you play you have no attachment to the outcome. You aren't too old or too adult to play, and you needn't treat it like a guilty pleasure when you indulge. Embrace play with all the abandon of a child—throw yourself into it and don't look back. It's good for you.

The Play of Art. Discover your own brand of play. For many of us, the impulse is to gravitate toward something we enjoy and excel at. But the very nature of play is to explore, to innovate, to be creative, and to experience anew. Pick up a tool. Take a class at a home-supply center and build something. Arm yourself with a paintbrush, a camera, a chisel, a quilting needle. Learn a craft. The mind devises, but the hand itself thinks, designs, knows. Find the flow in focused craftsmanship. Explore art, music, reading. Or take a mental break at work and throw paper airplanes or doodle caricatures. Let your imagination run free.

Primal Thrills. The urge to explore the limits of our minds, bodies, and environment is as natural as it is stirring. There's a certain thrill in testing your nerves, and when you're in the heady risk of action, time stops and you become raw awareness. We are factory-wired to want to explore our limits and our world in general, and if our thirst for adventure is constantly suppressed, we become bored and develop a sense of detached fatigue. Adrenaline rushes allow you to return to ordinary life refreshed and appreciative of simple pleasures. Whatever you choose to do, do it safely, with respect for the activity and your abilities—or lack thereof—and enjoy the heightened experience of knowing you are alive.

AUTHOR'S NOTE

I PROMISED IN THE INTRODUCTION that you'd get your hands dirty. I hope you've enjoyed the process of digging into our human past, sifting through the latest evolutionary evidence, and even grubbing in the rich and loamy soil of the garden. My intention through all this has been to help you engage the lens of evolutionary biology to show you how to turn on your "hidden genetic switches" and ultimately manifest greater joy, pleasure, fulfillment, and satisfaction in your life.

There are, of course, other topics we did not cover here, but the basic premise is always the same. When you honor the expectations of your hunter-gatherer genes and make those primal connections, you unlock your potential for increased health and happiness. In the final analysis, however, life is simply a matter of making choices. And in that regard, the real irony is that there are no right or wrong answers. Just choices—and, naturally—the effects of those choices.

I encourage you to allow the Primal Connection to become your personal story, to let it be told and unfold wherever you roam on your life journey. No matter the eventual trajectory, I trust you will find unprecedented health and discovery along the way. Go forth, embrace the full force of your inherent vitality, and live the best Primal life possible. Grok on!

Mark Sisson
Malibu, CA
November, 2012

NOTES

Recipe for Success

1. T. Hayashi, K. Murakami, "The Effects of Laughter on Post-Prandial Glucose Levels and Gene Expression in Type 2 Diabetic Patients," *Life Sciences Journal*, 85, 5-6 (July 2009): 185-7.

2. Y. Ohtsuka, N. Yabunaka, S. Takayama, "Shinrin-Yoku (Forest-Air Bathing and Walking) Effectively Decreases Blood Glucose Levels in Diabetic Patients," *International Journal of Biometeorology*, 41,3 (February 1998): 125-7.

3. N. Jutapakdeegul, S.O. Casalotti, P. Govitrapong, N. Kotchabhakdi, "Postnatal Touch Stimulation Acutely Alters Corticosterone Levels and Glucocorticoid Receptor Gene Expression in the Neonatal Rat," *Developmental Neuroscience*, 25, 1 (January-February 2003): 26-33.

4. K. Uvnas-Moberg, M. Petersson. "Oxytocin, A Mediator of Anti-Stress, Well-Being, Social Interaction, Growth, and Healing," *Zeitschrift für Psychosomatische Medizin und Psychotherapie*, 51, 1 (2005): 57-80.

5. G.S. Liu, H.E. Tsai, W.T. Weng, et al, "Systemic Pro-Opiomelanocortin Expression Induces Melanogenic Differentiation and Inhibits Tumor Angiogenesis in Established Mouse Melanoma," *Human Gene Therapy*, 22, 3 (March 14, 2011): 325-35.

6. S.V. Ramagopalan, A. Heger, et al, "A ChIP-seq Defined Genome-Wide Map of Vitamin D Receptor Binding: Associations With Disease and Evolution," *Genome Research*, 20 (October 2010): 1352-1360.

7. K. Berridge, e-mail to author on October 15, 2012.

8. N. Wade, "Eden? Maybe. But Where's the Apple Tree?" *New York Times* (April 30, 2009) Science Section.

The Inner Connection

1. A. Williams, "Friends of a Certain Age: Why Is It Hard to Make Friends Over 30?" *The New York Times* (July 13, 2012) Fashion Section.

2. D.G. Myers, "The Powers and Perils of Intuition," *Psychology Today* (November 1, 2002). http://www.psychologytoday.com/articles/200212/the-powers-and-perils-intuition.

3. R. Wolff, *Original Wisdom: Stories of an Ancient Way of Knowing* (Rochester, VT: Inner Traditions International, 2001).

4. B. Dehghan, E. Enjedani, F.A. Meybodi, S. Sadeghi, "The Study of Immediate, Unconscious, and Conscious Thought Condition in the Post Choice Satisfaction: A Replicated Study," *Procedia—Social and Behavioral Sciences*, 30 (2011): 1201-1204.

5. A. Dijksterhuis, T. Meurs, "Where Creativity Resides: The Generative Power of Unconscious Thought," *Consciousness and Cognition* 15, 1 (March 2006): 135-146.

6. M.E. McCullough, "The Forgiveness Instinct," *Greater Good: The Science of a Meaningful Life* (Spring 2008) http://greatergood.berkeley.edu/article/item/forgiveness_instinct.

7. N. Wolchover, "Why Humans Prevailed Over Neanderthals," *Discovery News* (June 5, 2012) http://news.discovery.com/history/humans-neanderthals-120605.html.

The Body Connection

1. W.J. Cromie, "Of Hugs and Hormones: Lack of Touch Puts Kids Out of Touch," *The Harvard University Gazette* (June 11, 1998).

2. K.M. Grewen, S.S. Girdler, J. Amico, K.C. Light, "Effects of Partner Support on Resting Oxytocin, Cortisol, Norepinephrine, and Blood Pressure Before and After Warm Partner Contact," *Psychosomatic Medicine*, 67, 4 (July 1, 2005): 531-538.

3. N. Dworkin-McDaniel, "Touching Makes You Healthier," *CNN.com* (January 5, 2011). http://www.cnn.com/2011/HEALTH/01/05/touching.makes.you.healthier.health/index.html.

4. T. Field, M. Hernandez-Reif, M. Diego, S. Schanberg, C. Kuhn, "Cortisol Decreases and Serotonin and Dopamine Increase Following Massage Therapy," *International Journal of Neuroscience*, 115, 10 (October 2005): 1397-1413.

5. T. Field, M. Hernandez-Reif, M.Diego, S. Schanberg, C. Kuhn, "Cortisol Decreases and Serotonin and Dopamine Increase Following Massage Therapy."

6. N. Dworkin-McDaniel, "Touching Makes You Healthier," *CNN.com.*

7. B. Leuner, E.R. Glasper, E. Gould, "Sexual Experience Promotes Adult Neurogenesis in the Hippocampus Despite an Initial Elevation in Stress Hormones," *Public Library of Science*, 5, 7 (July 14, 2010): e11597.

8. M.H. Rapaport, P. Schettler, C. Bresee, "A Preliminary Study of the Effects of a Single Session of Swedish Massage on Hypothalamic-Pituitary-Adrenal and Immune Function in Normal Individuals," *The Journal of Alternative and Complementary Medicine*, 16, 10 (September 1, 2010): 1-10.

9. B. Holmes, "Achilles Tendon Is Key to Evolution of Human Running," *New Scientist* (April 1, 2010) http://www.newscientist.com/article/dn18728-achilles-tendon-is-key-to-evolution-of-human-running.html.

10. F.M. Painter, "Forward Head Posture Page," *Chiro.org* (blog). Updated April 2, 2012, http://www.chiro.org/LINKS/Forward_Head_Posture.shtml.

11. R. Sakakibara, K. Tsunoyama, et al, "Influence of Body Position on Defecation in Humans," *LUTS: Lower Urinary Tract Symptoms*, 2, 1 (Janurary 11, 2010): 16-21.

12. E. Barclay, "For Best Toilet Health: Squat or Sit?" *NPR* (September 28, 2012) http://www.npr.org/blogs/health/2012/09/20/161501413/for-best-toilet-health-squat-or-sit; D. Sikirov, "Management of Hemorrhoids: A New Approach," *Israel Journal of Medical Sciences* (1987): 23, 284-286.

13. D. Sikirov, "Comparison of Straining During Defecation in Three Positions," *Digestive Diseases and* Sciences, 48, 7 (July 2003): 1201-1205.

14. C. Cotman, N. Berchtold, "Exercise: A Behavioral Intervention to Enhance Brain Health and Plasticity," *Trends in Neurosciences*, 25, 6 (June 2002): 295–301

15. Ibid.

16. O. Judson, "Stand Up While You Read This!" *The New York Times* (February 23, 2010) http://opinionator.blogs.nytimes.com/2010/02/23/stand-up-while-you-read-this/.

17. T. Yates, et al, "Self-Reported Sitting Time and Markers of Inflammation, Insulin Resistance, and Adiposity," *American Journal of Preventative Medicine*, 42, 1 (January 2012): 1-7.

18. A. Bankston, "Office-Dwellers Stand Up to 'Sitting Disease,'" *Star Tribune* (January 27, 2012). http://www.startribune.com/local/138174639.html?refer=y.

19. S.J. Colcombe, et al, "Aerobic Fitness Reduces Brain Tissue Loss in Aging Humans," *The Journals of Gerontology, Series A, Biological Sciences and Medical Sciences*, 58, 2 (February 2003): 176-180.

20. L.E. Hill, S.K. Droste, et al, "Voluntary Exercise Alters GABA(A) Receptor Subunit and Glutamic Acid Decarboxylase-67 Gene Expression in the Rat Forebrain," *Journal of* Psychopharmacology, 24, 5 (May 2010): 745-756.

21. C.C. Streeter, et al, "Effects of Yoga Versus Walking on Mood, Anxiety, and Brain GABA Levels: A Randomized Controlled MRS Study," *The Journal of Alternative and Complementary Medicine*, 16, 11 (November 2010): 1145-1152.

The Nature Connection

1. A. Stevens, *The Two Million-Year-Old Self* (College Station, TX: Texas A&M University Press, 1993).

2. S. Kumar, K. Kriegstein, K. Friston, T. Griffeths, "Features Versus Feelings: Dissociable Representations of the Acoustic Features and Valence of Aversive Sounds," *The Journal of Neuroscience*, 32, 41 (October 10, 2012): 14184-14192.

3. D. March, "Nature's Sights, Sounds Ease Pain During Bone Marrow Extraction," *The Johns Hopkins Gazette* (Oct. 18, 2010) http://gazette.jhu.edu/2010/10/18/nature%E2%80%99s-sights-sounds-ease-pain-during-bone-marrow-extraction/.

4. B.J. Park, Y. Tsunetsugu, T. Kasetani, T. Kagawa, Y. Miyazaki, "The Physiological Effects of Shinrin-Yoku (Taking in the Forest Atmosphere or Forest Bathing): Evidence From Field Experiments in 24 Forests Across Japan," *Environmental Health and Preventative Medicine*, 15, 1 (January 2010): 18-26.

5. Q. Li, "Effect of Forest Bathing Trips on Human Immune Function," *Environmental Health and Preventative Medicine*, 15, 1 (January 2010): 9-17.

6. M. Roberts, "The Touchy-Feely (but Totally Scientific!) Methods of Wallace J. Nichols," *Outside Magazine* (November 8, 2011) http://www.outsideonline.com/outdoor-adventure/nature/The-Touchy-Feely-But-Totally-Scientific-Methods-Of-Wallace-J-Nichols.html?page=all.

7. Ibid.

8. F. Soyka, *The Ion Effect* (Toronto, Canada: Lester and Orpen Limited, 1977): 145-146.

9. D. Reid, *The Tao of Health, Sex, and Longevity: A Modern Practical Guide to the Ancient Way* (New York: Touchstone Publishing, 1989).

10. C. Ober, M. Zucker, *Earthing: The Most Important Health Discovery Ever?* (Laguna Beach, CA: Basic Health Publications, Inc., 2010).

11. Ibid.

12. Ibid.

13. P.H. Kahn Jr., et al, "A Plasma Display Window?—The Shifting Baseline Problem in a Technologically Mediated Natural World," *Journal of Environmental Psychology*, 28, 2 (May 8, 2008): 192-199.

14. "Dogs That Changed the World: What Caused the Domestication of Wolves?" *PBS.org* http://www.pbs.org/wnet/nature/episodes/dogs-that-changed-the-world/what-caused-the-domestication-of-wolves/1276/.

15. N.A. Shevchuk, S. Radoja, "Possible Stimulation of Anti-Tumor Immunity Using Repeated Cold Stress: A Hypothesis," *Infectious Agents and Cancer* 2, 20 (November 12, 2007); regarding muscle recovery: C. Bleakley, S. McDonough, E. Gardner, G.D. Baxter, J.T. Hopkins, G.W. Davison, "Cold-Water Immersion (Cryotherapy) for Preventing and Treating Muscle Soreness After Exercise," *The Cochrane Library*, 2 (February 15, 2012).

16. W. Davis, *The Wayfinders: Why Ancient Wisdom Matters in the Modern World* (Toronto: House of Anansi Press, Inc., 2009).

17. R. Louv, *The Nature Principle* (Chapel Hill, NC: Algonquin Books, 2011).

18. Hui-Mei Chen, Hung-Ming Tu, Chaang-Iuan Ho, "Exploring Dimensions of Attitudes Toward Horticultural Activities," *HortScience*, 45(7), (July 2010). http://hortsci.ashspublications.org/content/45/7/1120.abstract.

19. A.E. Van Den Berg, et all, "Allotment Gardening and Health: A Comparative Survey Among Allotment Gardeners and Their Neighbors Without an Allotment," *Environmental Health*, 9, 74 (2010) http://www.ehjournal.net/content/9/1/74

20. A.J. Sommerfeld, T.M. Waliczek, J.M. Zajicek, "Growing Minds: Evaluating the Effect of Gardening on Quality of Life and Physical Activity Level of Older Adults." *HortTechnology*, 20, (2010) http://horttech.ashspublications.org/content/20/4/705.abstract.

The Rhythm Connection

1. T. Saitoa, R. Okamotoa, T. Harituniansa, J. O'Kellya, et al., "Novel Gemini Vitamin D3 Analogs Have Potent Antitumor Activity," *The Journal of Steroid Biochemistry and Molecular Biology*, 112, 1-3 (November 2008): 151-56.

2. K. Than, "Americans Are Info-Junkies," *TechNewsDaily*, (December 14, 2009) http://www.technewsdaily.com/16-americans-are-info-junkies-.html.

3. M. Richtel, "Attached to Technology and Paying a Price," *The New York Times* (June 6, 2010). Technology section.

4. T.F. Juster, et al., "Changing Times of American Youth: 1981-2003," *Institute for Social Research, University of Michigan*. Child Development Supplement (2004), http://www.ns.umich.edu/Releases/2004/Nov04/teen_time_report.pdf.

5. V. Rideout, et al, "Generation M: Media in the Lives of 8-18 Year-Olds," *The Henry J. Kaiser Family Foundation* (2005). http://www.kff.org/entmedia/entmedia030905pkg.cfm.

6. M. Richtel, "Attached to Technology and Paying a Price," *The New York Times* (June 6, 2010) http://www.nytimes.com/2010/06/07/technology/07brain.html?pagewanted=all

7. "The Sourcebook for Teaching Science," California State University, Northridge. http://www.csun.edu/science/health/docs/tv&health.html.

8. "Watching TV Linked to Post Traumatic Stress Disorder," University of Bolton. (April 1, 2009) http://www.bolton.ac.uk/News/News-Articles/2009/apr2009-2.aspx

9. *Jakob Nielsen's Alert Box* (blog). http://www.useit.com/alertbox/page-abandonment-time.html.

10. T. Tamkins, "Drop That BlackBerry! Multitasking May Be Harmful," *CNN.com* (August 25, 2009) http://www.cnn.com/2009/HEALTH/08/25/multitasking.harmful/index.html?iref=allsearch.

11. J. Hamilton, "Think You're Multitasking? Think Again," *NPR.org* (October 2, 2008). http://www.npr.org/templates/story/story.php?storyId=95256794

12. Regarding metabolic syndrome: "Moderate Exercise Cuts Rate of Metabolic Syndrome," DukeHealth.org (Dec. 17, 2007). http://www.dukehealth.org/health_library/news/10205; regarding breast cancer: S.A. Adams,

et al., "Association of Physical Activity with Hormone Receptor Status: The Shanghai Breast Cancer Study," *Cancer Epidemiology, Biomarkers & Prevention*, 15 (June 2006); regarding cardiovascular and mortality: J. Myers, et al., "Exercise Capacity and Mortality among Men Referred for Exercise Testing," *New England Journal of Medicine* (March 14, 2002): 793-801

13. D. Avni-Babad, "Routine and Feelings of Safety, Confidence, and Well-Being," *British Journal of Psychology*, 102, 2 (March 11, 2011): 223-44.

14. M. Csikszentmihalyi, *Finding Flow: The Psychology of Engagement with Everyday Life*, (New York: Basic Books, 1997).

15. M. Csikszentmihalyi, "Finding Flow," *Psychology Today* (July 1, 1997). http://www.psychologytoday.com/articles/199707/finding-flow.

16. M. Csikszentmihalyi, *Finding Flow: The Psychology of Optimal Experience*.

17. Sat Bir S. Khalsa, et al., "Yoga Ameliorates Performance Anxiety and Mood Disturbance in Young Professional Musicians," *Applied Psychophysiology and Biofeedback*, 34, 4 (December 2009): 278-89.

The Social Connection

1. *Early Human Kinship: From Sex to Social Reproduction*, N. J. Allen, H. Callan, R. Dunbar, W. James, Eds. (West Sussex, U.K.: Blackwell-Wiley, 2011); S. Mithen, *After the Ice: A Global Human History 20,000-5000 BC*, (Cambridge: Harvard University Press, 2003).

2. *Early Human Kinship: From Sex to Social Reproduction*, N.J. Allen, H. Callan, R. Dunbar, W. James, Eds.

3. T. Ingold, "On the Social Relations of the Hunter-gatherer Band," *The Cambridge Encyclopedia of Hunters and Gatherers*, Richard B. Lee, Richard Daly, Eds., (Cambridge: Cambridge University Press, 1999).

4. Regarding motor skill retention: A.S. Buchman, et al., "Association Between Late-Life Social Activity and Motor Decline in Older Adults," *Archives of Internal Medicine*, 169, 12 (June 22, 2009): 1139-46; regarding cancer survival: C.H. Kroenke, "Social Networks, Social Support, and Survival After Breast Cancer Diagnosis," *Journal of Clinical Oncology* 24, 7 (March 1, 2006): 1105-11; regarding immune response: S.D. Pressman, et al., "Loneliness, Social Network Size, and Immune Response to Influenza Vaccination in College Freshmen," *Health Psychology*, 24, 3 (July 2005): 348; regarding memory preservation: K.A. Ertel, et al., "Effects of Social Integration on Preserving Memory Function in a Nationally Representative U.S. Elderly Population," *American Journal of Public Health* 98, 7 (May 29, 2008): 1215-20; regarding longevity: L.C. Giles, "Effect of Social Networks on 10 Year Survival in Very Old Australians: the Australian Longitudinal Study of Aging," *Journal of Epidemiology & Community Health*, 59 (2005).

5. Regarding Alzheimer's: R.S. Wilson, et al., "Loneliness and Risk of Alzheimer's Disease," *Archives of General Psychiatry*, 64, 2 (2007): 234-40; regarding heart disease: K. Orth-Gomer, et al., "Lack of Social Support and Incidence of Coronary Heart Disease in Middle-Aged Swedish Men," *Psychosomatic Medicine*, 55, 1 (Jan-Feb, 1993): 37-43.

6. J. Holt-Lunstad, T.B. Smith, J.B. Layton, "Social Relationships and Mortality Risk: A Meta-analytic Review," *PLOS Medicine* (July 27, 2010). http://www.plosmedicine.org/article/info:doi/10.1371/journal.pmed.1000316

7. L. F. Berkman, S. L. Syme, "Social Networks, Host Resistance, and Mortality: A Nine-Year Follow-Up Study of Alameda County Residents," *American Journal of Epidemiology*, 109, 2 (July 25, 1978): 186-204.

8. E.M. Friedman, "Sleep Quality, Social Well-Being, Gender, and Inflammation: An Integrative Analysis in a National Sample," *Annals of the New York Academy of Sciences*, 1231 (August 2011): 23-34.

9. R. Dunbar, "Neocortex Size as a Constraint on Group Size in Primates," *Journal of Human Evolution*, 22 (December 1992): 20, 469-93; R. Dunbar, "Kinship in Biological Perspective," *Early Human Kinship: From Sex to Social Reproduction*, N.J. Allen, H. Callan, R. Dunbar, W. James, Eds. (West Sussex, U.K.: Blackwell-Wiley, 2011): 131-50.

10. R. Dunbar, "Neocortex Size as a Constraint on Group Size in Primates," *Journal of Human Evolution*, 22.

11. M. Connelly, "More Americans Sense a Downside to an Always Plugged-In Existence," *The New York Times* (June 6, 2010). Technology section.

12. L. Jaremka, et al., "What Makes Us Feel the Best Also Makes Us Feel the Worst: The Emotional Impact of Independent and Interdependent Experiences," *Self and Identity* 10 (March 23, 2010): 44-63.

13. G.J. Stephens, "Speaker-listener Neural Coupling Underlies Successful Communication," *PNAS* 107, 32 (July 26, 2010). http://www.pnas.org/content/early/2010/07/13/1008662107.abstract

14. D.J. Hruschka, et al., "Shared Norms and Their Explanation for the Social Clustering of Obesity," *American Journal of Public Health*, 101, Suppl.1 (May 9, 2011): S295-300.

15. J. Gokee LaRose, T.M. Leahey, B.M. Weinberg, R. Kumar, R.R. Wing, "Young Adults' Performance in a Low Intensity Weight Loss Campaign," *Obesity* 20, 11 (November 2012): 2314-6.

16. D. Marron, "Memories Are a Durable Investment," *The Christian Science Monitor* (blog: May 1, 2012). http://www.csmonitor.com/Business/Donald-Marron/2012/0501/Memories-are-a-durable-investment.

17. Ibid.

18. C. Sedikides, et al., "Nostalgia: Past, Present, and Future," *Current Directions in Psychological Science*, 17, 5 (Oct. 2008): 304-07.

19. P. Arnstein, et al., "From Chronic Pain Patient to Peer: Benefits and Risks of Volunteering," *Pain Management Nursing*, 3, 3 (September 2002): 94-103.

20. N. Krause, et al., "Providing Support to Others and Well-Being in Later Life," *Journal of Gerontology*, 47, 5 (September 1992): 301-11.

21. *Handbook of Mind-Body Medicine for Primary Care*, ed. D. Moss, et al., (Thousand Oaks, CA: Sage Publications, 2003).

22. P. Arnstein, "From Chronic Pain Patient to Peer: Benefits and Risks of Volunteering," *Pain Management Nursing*, 3, 3 (Sept. 2002): 94-103.

23. Emory University. "Compassion Meditation May Improve Physical And Emotional Responses To Psychological Stress." *ScienceDaily*, 7 Oct. 2008. http://www.sciencedaily.com/releases/2008/10/081007172902.htm

The Play Connection

1. P. Sims, "The Montessori Mafia," *The Wall Street Journal* (April 5, 2011). Review section.

2. B. Elgin, "Managing Google's Idea Factory," *Businessweek.com* (Oct. 2, 2005). http://www.businessweek.com/stories/2005-10-02/managing-googles-idea-factory

3. "The Weight of the Nation," *HBO* (website). http://theweightofthenation.hbo.com/films/main-films/Consequences.

4. Ilanit Gordon, et. al., "Oxytocin and the Development of Parenting in Humans," *Biological Psychiatry*, 68, 4 (Aug. 15, 2010): 377-82.

5. "Use It or Lose It: Mind Games Help Healthy Older People Too," *BioMed Central* (March 27, 2012). http://www.biomedcentral.com/presscenter/pressreleases/20120327

6. D. Jopp, C. Rott, "Adaptation in Very Old Age: Exploring the Role of Resources, Beliefs, and Attitudes for Centenarians' Happiness," *Psychology and Aging*, 21, 2 (2006): 266-280

7. Marian Vanhaeren, et al., "Middle Paleolithic Shell Beads in Israel and Algeria," *Science Magazine*, 12, 5781 (June 23, 2006): 1785-88.

8. Stuart Brown, *Play: How It Shapes the Brain, Opens the Imagination, and Invigorates the Soul* (New York: Penguin Group, 2009).

9. Clive Gamble, "Kinship and Material Culture: Archeological Implications of the Human Global Diaspora," *Early Human Kinship: From Sex to Social Reproduction*, eds. N.J. Allen, H. Callan, R. Dunbar, W. James (West Sussex, UK: Blackwell Publishing Ltd, 2011).

10. "Weaving Traditional Arts into the Fabric of Community Health," *Alliance for California Traditional Arts* (Oct. 2011). http://www.actaonline.org/sites/default/files/images/docs/briefing.pdf.

11. P. Ghosh, "Oldest Musical Instrument Found," *BBC News* (June 25, 2009). http://news.bbc.co.uk/2/hi/science/nature/8117915.stm.

12. G. Marcus, G. Miller, "Did Humans Invent Music?" *The Atlantic* (April 16, 2012). http://m.theatlantic.com/entertainment/archive/2012/04/did-humans-invent-music/255945/

13. N. Uedo, et al., "Reduction in Salivary Cortisol Level by Music Therapy During Colonoscopic Examination," *Hepato-gastroenterology*, 51, 56 (Mar-Apr 2004): 451-3; T. Yamamoto, et al., "Effects of Pre-exercise Listening to Slow and Fast Rhythm Music on Supramaximal Cycle Performance and Selected Metabolic Variables," *Archives of Physiology and Biochemistry* 3, 3 (July 2003): 211-14; C. Conrad, et al., "Overture for Growth Hormone: Requiem for Interleukin-6?" *Critical Care Medicine* 35, 12 (December 2007).

14. N.K. Dess, "Music On the Mind," *Psychology Today* (September 1, 2000). http://www.psychologytoday.com/articles/200008/music-the-mind; "Music Training Enhances Brainstem Sensitivity to Speech Sounds, Neuroscientist Says," *Science Daily* (February 22, 2010). http://www.sciencedaily.com/releases/2010/02/100220184327.htm

15. D. Ackerman, *A Natural History of the Senses* (New York: Random House, 1990).

response
  emotional, 46
  vs. reaction, 46
responsibility, 44–47
  Feed the Habit, 47
  pleasure and, 36
reward system, for survival, 22
rhythm of life, 137
Ridley, Matt, 34
risk, 225–226
  calculated, 227–228
risk-versus-reward factor, 228
rituals
  for ancestors, 203

  for emotional closure, 63
rhythm of, 178–179
Rogers, Will, 98
Roosevelt, Eleanor, 224
RSS feeds, 165
Ruebush, Mary, 129
running
  Achilles tendon and, 86
  barefoot, 82, 83, 88
Ryan, Frank, 173

S

sacrifice, vs. selfishness, 49
Sagan, Carl, 218
Sahlins, Marshall, 66, 69
Sanders, Scott Russell, 117
sanitation. *See also* dirt
  immune system and, 125–127
satisfaction, meaning of, 11
scarcity, 35–36
  vs. abundance, 15, 21
Schultheis, Rob, 229
SCN. *See* suprachiasmatic
  nucleus

season, sleep habits and, 149
sedentary lifestyle, 100–102
  vitamin D and, 153
segmented sleep, 148
self-analysis, 40–42
self-awareness, 42
self-control, 44
self-development, 64–65
  Feed the Habit, 65
  play for, 221
self-evaluation, of present vs.
  desired life, 47

self-interest, acting against, 43
Selfish Gene, The (Dawkins), 48
selfishness, 48–50
  Feed the Habit, 49–50
  play and, 216
  vs. sacrifice, 49
self talk, 40–42, 43, 44
  kinder, 50
  negative, 62–63
Sellers, Bill, 86
sensory awareness, 27, 28
  exercising senses, 116
  intuition and, 56–59
  nature and, 109–111
  touch and, 74–79
serotonin, 21, 25, 130
  sunlight and, 141, 150
sex, touch and, 78
Shepard, Paul, 191
shoes
  brands of, 83–85
  going barefoot and, 80, 82–83
  Vibram FiveFingers, 83–84
sight, 109
Silberbauer, George B., 121
silence, 183–186

Simple Abundance
  (Breathnach), 69
single-tasking, mindful, 170–172
sitting, 100–102
  breaks from, 102
  vs. squatting, 95–97
skin
  light sensitivity of, 144
  touch and, 74–79
  vitamin D and, 152
skin cancer, vitamin D
  deficiencies and, 153
skin color, vitamin D, sunshine,
  and, 154
Skinner, B.F., 29
slacklining, 233–234
sleep, 139
  bedroom and, 143–144
  bi- or polyphasic, 148
  difficulties with, 139–140
  historical information about,
    147–148
  optimal amounts of, 148–149
  REM and non-REM, 144–145
  seasonal sunlight and, 149
  social connections and, 193
sleep hacks, 151–152
sleep maintenance insomnia, 148
sleep masks, 150
Slow Food movement, 176
slowing down, energy output
  and, 175–186
Slow Living movement, 176, 178
smell, 109, 110–111
social circle, 50–52. *See also*
  friends; Social Connection
  obesity in, 201
Social Connection, 17–18,
  189–209

THE PRIMAL CONNECTION

PRIMAL
BLUEPRINT

Other books by Primal Blueprint Publishing

MARK SISSON

The Primal Blueprint: *Reprogram your genes for effortless weight loss, vibrant health, and boundless energy*

The Primal Blueprint 21-Day Total Body Transformation: *A step-by-step gene reprogramming action plan*

The Primal Blueprint 90-Day Journal: *A Personal Experiment (n=1)*

COOKBOOKS BY MARK SISSON AND JENNIFER MEIER

The Primal Blueprint Cookbook: *Primal, low carb, paleo, grain-free, dairy-free and gluten-free meals*

The Primal Blueprint Quick and Easy Meals: *Delicous, Primal-approved meals you can make in under 30 minutes*

The Primal Blueprint Healthy Sauces, Dressings, and Toppings: *Plus rubs, dips, marinades and other easy ways to transform basic natural foods into Primal masterpieces*

OTHER AUTHORS
Rich Food, Poor Food: *The Ultimate Grocery Purchasing System (GPS)*, by Mira Calton, CN, and Jayson Calton, Ph.D.